The Medical Garden

Geoffrey Marks
and William K. Beatty

THE

MEDICAL

GARDEN

ILLUSTRATED

CHARLES SCRIBNER'S SONS
New York

Picture Credits

Académie Nationale de Médicine. No. 20

Annals of Internal Medicine 11:1635, 1938. No. 13

La Farmacia Storica ed Artistica Italiana (Milan: Edizioni Vittoria, 1934). No. 4

Fritz Johannessohn, *Chinin in der Allgemeinpraxis* (Amsterdam: Bureau tot Bevordering van het Kinine-Gebruik, 1930). Nos. 10, 11

Journal of the American Pharmaceutical Association, April 1929. No. 3

Gustav Kunze, *Pharmaceutische Waarenkunde,* vol. 2 (Eisenach: Bärecke, 1830-1834). No. 15

Adam Lonicerus, *Kreuterbuch* (Ulm: Matthew Wagner, 1679). No. 17

Pietro Mattioli, *I Discorsi . . . nelli sei Libri di Pedacio Dioscoride . . .* (Venice: Valgrisius, 1581). No. 14

Medical and Biological Illustration, 18: 62-70, 1968, Nos. 1, 5, 6

Musée du Val-de-Grace. No. 21

Northwestern University Medical Library, Nos. 2, 7, 8, 9, 18, 19, 22

Salerno 1:33, January/February, 1967. No. 16

Scientific Monthly (now *Science*) 57:19, 1943. No. 12

This book published simultaneously in the United States of America and in Canada— Copyright under the Berne Convention

A - 9.71 [H]

Printed in the United States of America
Library of Congress Catalog Card Number 74-167777
SBN 684-12383-5

For Katherine True Becker

Contents

Illustrations

Preface

This book traces the development of seven drugs, all originally derived from plant forms, all in wide use today. Their stories cover the manner in which each plant was used, the gradual growth of knowledge about its effectiveness, and the often exciting unfolding of the scientific work that secured its use and dosage as a drug in modern medicine. The men and events involved in the growth of this knowledge present a lively picture of folklore turning to science.

All seven drugs can do tremendous good. But they must be used with care. Uncontrolled doses can prove extremely dangerous, even fatal.

Opium has many medicinal uses. Among them, more often than not in its modern medical form—morphine, are the reduction of pain, the control of contractions in certain conditions, such as severe diarrhea, and in childbirth. However, every day's newspaper tells of deaths resulting from the misuse of morphine or the use of heroin, another derivative of opium. Unfortunately, the amount that can be tolerated varies enormously with the individual and the situation. In addition, individuals "on" opium and its derivatives become addicted and find themselves dependent upon greater and greater doses. The end of the road is death, often in deplorable circumstances.

Cocaine was established as one of the first local anesthetics, especially useful in eye surgery. It was believed by no less an authority than Sigmund Freud that cocaine was a nonaddictive substitute for morphine, but it turned out to be as entrapping as its predecessor. Used to excess, it can cause overexcitement, an abnormally rapid fluttering of the heart, fainting, and even convulsions and collapse.

Quinine is derived from a bark which, in powdered form, has been used for some centuries to control malaria. But quinine too has its problem side. Doses considered necessary to the reduction of fever can cause ringing in the ears, headache, nausea, dizziness, and disturbed vision, all symptoms of poisoning.

Aspirin, known as the "safest" remedy, is widely used for headaches, rheumatism, and fever, but overdoses cause deaths among adults and children each year.

Colchicine not only relieves the pain of gout but also increases the response of cancer cells to x-ray treatment. However, colchicine can cause vomiting, bloody diarrhea, delirium, and shock.

Digitalis is essential in certain types of heart conditions, but the problem of determining a proper dosage, different for each individual, kept doctors from prescribing it for many years. Even today a patient under medical "control" can become overdigitalized, with serious consequences.

Penicillin is a recognized, almost universal lifesaver. But some people are or become allergic to it, and there have even been cases in which individuals drinking milk from a cow treated with penicillin have had violent reactions. Then too, certain bacteria can build resistance to penicillin. Consequently, overuse or unnecessary use of penicillin may render it powerless when it is most needed.

These drugs, indeed most drugs, have this in common: proper use can be highly beneficial; misuse, or abuse, is dangerous and sometimes fatal.

One

"The Plant
of Good and Evil"   ✌✌
⌐ Opium

THE JUICE OF
THE WHITE POPPY

Opium is the dried juice or sap of the unripe seedpod of *Papaver somniferum*—the white poppy. Today it is better known in medical circles as *morphine,* which is the principal alkaloid derived from opium. Heroin, a more potent form of morphine, is a notorious narcotic, whose importation, production, and sale are illegal in the United States.

The white poppy has grown wild in Asia Minor since earliest days. It has also been found in its native state in waste places and in the wheat fields of England. But there does not seem to be a time when it was not cultivated commercially. Such cultivation began in Asia Minor. It has spread to Turkey, Persia (Iran), Bulgaria, Yugoslavia, North Africa, India, China, and Mexico (where it is raised illegally). An attempt to produce opium in the United States failed. The reason given for this failure was high labor costs. These may have contributed, but climate was certainly another factor. *Papaver somniferum* only yields enough latex (sap) to make the production of opium profitable when it is grown in warm, sunny climes. Climate, as much as cheap labor, was responsible for successful opium cultivation in China, India, and other tropical and subtropical areas.

The white or opium poppy is a member of a large botanical family that includes some 250 species. A number of these are at home in the temperate regions of the northern hemisphere where gardeners have bred a variety of forms. All poppies yield some of the milky juice that is dried to produce opium. But it is the

3

white poppy that gives the best quality of opium, with a morphine yield running as high as 10-20 percent.

The Asia Minor opium plant has had a spectacular and widespread influence on history. Battles have been fought to gain control of its sleep-producing juice; nations have been retarded by the lure of its dream-producing properties.

EARLY USE
OF OPIUM

What is probably the earliest record of the medical use of opium dates to the sixteenth century B.C. The Ebers papyrus, a medical treatise compiled at that time, instructs Egyptian mothers to use opium to quiet their babies. A century later the subjects of King Tutankhamen were taking a mixture of opium, coriander, wormwood, juniper, and honey as a cure for hangover.

But the use of opium as a means of escaping from reality began much earlier. Tablets that have come down from the Sumerians who lived in Babylon as far back as 4000 B.C. refer to the poppy as the plant of joy. About the same time, Stone Age lake dwellers in Switzerland were storing *cultivated* poppy seeds and seed heads in their living places. This suggests that the primitive inhabitants of Europe discovered the narcotic effect of opium before they learned to write and read.

Homer wrote his *Odyssey* around 1000 B.C. He speaks therein of the "drug, nepenthes, which gave forgetfulness of evil. Those who had drunk of this mixture did not shed a tear the whole day long, even though their mother or father were dead, even though a brother or beloved son had been killed before their eyes by the weapons of the enemy. . . ."[1] It seems likely that the potion consisted largely of opium.

The Greeks used the poppy in several ways. They sprinkled

the seeds, which do not contain opium, on their cakes. (We continue this practice today in bread, rolls, and pastries sprinkled with poppy seeds.) They boiled the entire plant to make a mild sleeping draught called *meconium*. Finally, they made opium from the juice of the unripe seed pod. They called the product *opos,* meaning "sap." It is, of course, from *opos* that the name *opium* comes.

Opium (in wine) was used as a poison as early as the fourth century B.C. when Cornelius Nepos arranged for doctors to give his father, Dionysius, an overdose of opium and "he died as though he slept himself to death."[2] In 399 B.C. Socrates, whose mind was rated the wisest and shrewdest in Athens, was convicted of impiety and the corruption of youth through his teaching. Custom of the day required him to take his own life. He selected hemlock, derived from a member of the carrot family. But it is clear that he recognized a choice between this and opium. About two centuries later, Hannibal, famous for crossing the Alps with his elephants, carried opium in his ring against an emergency. Then, at the beginning of the Christian era, Nero's mother Agrippina, second wife of the Emperor Claudius, put opium into the wine of her stepson Britannicus to clear the way to the imperial throne for her own son.

Turning to opium's medical history, in the fifth century B.C. Diagoras of Melos, a philosopher, was very much opposed to opium. He considered it better to bear pain than to take a drug upon which one might become dependent. This is the earliest recognition of the addictive properties of opium and its derivatives. Hippocrates, "the father of medicine" (460-357 B.C.), included opium among the powerful drugs, the use of which was to be discouraged.

By the end of the third century B.C., however, the Greek botanist Theophrastus, a student of Aristotle, was recommending poppy extract as an agent to induce vomiting and as an anticonvulsant. Herakleides of Tarentum was the first doctor to prescribe opium as a painkiller, notwithstanding the fact that he recognized that it was habit-forming. This was around 100 B.C. In A.D. 25 Cornelius Celsus was offering a "sory" for prevention of tooth decay. It consisted of poppy seed, pepper, and copper sulphate made into a paste. Celsus was loud in his praise of opium. Fifteen years later Pliny the Elder distinguished between pod-produced opium and the less effective meconium extracted from the whole plant. About the same time Scribonius Largus told how opium juice should be obtained from the seed pod. Then around A.D. 77 Pedanios Dioskorides (40-90) in turn described how the poppy pod should be slit and the juice collected. The method he outlined is still followed today.

The poppy plant is put in the ground in November. It flowers in April and May and the seed pod matures in June and July, a short time after the petals and stamen of the plant have fallen. Ripeness is determined by pressing the seed capsule. It is ripe when it turns pale under pressure. The capsule is slashed with multibladed knives, similar to those that were used in bloodletting. The capsule is scratched daily for six days. Cutting is generally done in the evening, and the sap, which thickens when it comes in contact with the air, is collected in the morning. The latex is scraped off with a small iron spoon shaped like a trowel. It is kept moist with spit, sweat, water, or oil to prevent the latex from sticking to it. When enough scrapings have accumulated, they are kneaded by hand into cakes, balls, or sticks. These are covered with poppy leaves and dried for several days.

In the first century A.D. Philon of Tarsus invented a cure-all which he called philonium. It consisted of opium, saffron, pyrethrum, euphorbium, henbane, spikenard, and other ingredients. It was so well accepted that it continued in use for centuries.

The second century produced Galen, who was to remain the supreme authority on medicine and pharmacology at least through the sixteenth century. His remedy for toothache involved black pepper, saffron, opium, carrot seeds, aniseed, and parsley seed.

The mixture was placed in the cavity of the offending tooth. Galen recognized that opium was valuable in the relief of a number of medical problems. Nonetheless he advised that it be used with caution. He had watched the Roman emperor Antoninus Pius become addicted to it.

The use of opium as a medicine, as a poison, and as a pleasure drug seems to have been largely localized. It made its appearance in Babylon, in prehistoric Switzerland, in Egypt, in Greece, in Rome, in Britain. But it was not regarded as an item of international trade. In England between the fifth and tenth centuries poppy sap was used externally for the treatment of sore eyes and taken internally for the cure of headache and sleeplessness. But its appearance there is not traceable to the Roman occupation.

The worldwide spread of opium must be laid at the wandering feet of the Prophet Mohammed. Mohammed is remembered as the founder of the Moslem faith. However, the real miracle for which he was responsible involved the welding of nomadic tribes of warriors and brigands into a compact Arabian nation. Mohammed died in A.D. 632. Within a century his followers had created an empire that stretched 5,000 miles from the Pyrenees dividing France and Spain in the west to the borders of India in the east.

The Koran, the book of Allah's revelations to Mohammed, forbade the drinking of wine. In obedience, the Moslems destroyed the vineyards wherever they went. But the Koran said nothing about the hard drugs such as opium and hashish. Both were adopted as a substitute for alcohol. Opium reached India and China by the tenth century. Its chief use in both countries was medicinal. Opium was used as a stimulant by a limited few. Opium eating and opium smoking on a broad scale was to come later.

A STANDARD
REMEDY

In India, opium became the standard remedy for a variety of problems ranging from dysentery to crying babies. It will be recalled that this use of opium to quiet babies had originated in Egypt twenty-five centuries earlier. It was to recur (unbeknownst to parents) in the United States in the nineteenth century when patent medicines (trademarked medical preparations) containing opium dominated the American drug market. Babies were actually turned into addicts by these "soothing syrups" represented as innocent tonics. The Pure Food and Drug Act of 1906 ended this practice.

The Moslems introduced opium wherever they went. This distribution of the beneficial but deadly drug was "rewarded" by a tragedy close to home. Ibn Sina (980-1037), or Avicenna as he became known to posterity, was an eminent philosopher, scientist, statesman, and poet, in addition to being named by his contemporaries "the Prince of Physicians." His life was one of unbelievable accomplishments. But it came to an end in 1037 when he was fifty-seven, after many years of overindulgence, including too much wine, which he was forbidden as a Moslem, and of attacks of colic. During his final illness one of his servants, who had already robbed him, tried to kill him by introducing into his medicine a great quantity of opium, which was of course readily available to Moslems. The attempt failed. Avicenna ultimately gave up all medicines, saying, "the manager who used to manage me is incapable of managing me any longer, so there is no use trying to cure my illness."[3]

Hua T'o (*ca.* 190-265) was the most famous surgeon in

Chinese history. His fame rests both on his great surgical skill and his use of anesthetics. He produced anesthesia with an "effervescing powder" in wine. Word of his work in anesthesia was brought to the West by Arab doctors a thousand years later. Within another one hundred years, the medical school of the University of Salerno in southern Italy was teaching about surgical sleeping draughts. One of these contained opium, henbane, mulberry juice, hemlock, mandragora, and ivy. A list of drugs passing in quantity through an Italian customhouse prepared about the same time includes opium.

By the fifteenth century Venice had taken control of the drug and spice trade. Drugs went from Venice over the Alps into Germany. Galleys carried them by sea to Bruges in Belgium and sometimes directly to London or Southampton. These galleys called at such ports as Pola, Corfu, Alicante, Almeria, Cadiz, and Lisbon. Opium was among the drugs distributed to all these ports. Opium had at length become an item of trade.

In fact, opium was one of the commodities Columbus hoped to bring back from the Indies when he sailed west but found the wrong Indies. So it was left to Portuguese ships sailing round the Cape of Good Hope to capture the Eastern trade. The opium they brought back was mostly used as medicine, seldom as a pleasure drug. Opium would not become a serious social problem until some centuries later.

Theophrastus Bombastus von Hohenheim (1493-1541), better known as Paracelsus, was born at Einsiedeln, Switzerland, the son of a doctor. Paracelsus's claim to fame as a physician was twofold. Like his contemporary Girolamo Fracastoro (1483-1553) of Verona, who was among the first to point toward the existence of disease germs, Paracelsus challenged the medical teaching that had been accepted for over a thousand years. He later came to be regarded as the father of medical chemistry.

Paracelsus studied medicine in Italy at the University of Ferrara. In his later writings, he stated that his university years were disappointing to him because the teaching was so theoretical. His youth had been spent in the fields, in the woods, in the mines, and among his father's patients. He had learned science from experience rather than books.

"Paracelsus at this time was already too much of a personality to let himself be forced into the traditional pattern. If the universities could not teach him what he wanted to learn, other people would. Who? Barber-surgeons, old women, craftsmen, miners, abbots, scholars, or laymen. What difference did it make? You must learn from any source that you can tap. He realized, however, that he would have to travel, and from Italy he set out on a journey which with short interruptions was to continue all his life and which only death brought to an end."[4]

His travels covered southern Europe, the British Isles, much of Scandinavia, the Baltic States, and the Balkans. He also visited Rhodes, Samos, Constantinople, Crete, and Alexandria. He practiced medicine as he went, seeing a great variety of diseases. It was then that he developed his personal approach to treatment, which involved the use of specific drugs, including opium which he employed frequently. His approach was in direct opposition to that of the followers of Galen, the great Greek physician of the second century A.D. They advocated compound remedies with up to twenty or more ingredients. Paracelsus believed that in such remedies the various drugs cancelled each other out.

In 1527 Paracelsus was offered and accepted the post of municipal physician in the Swiss city of Basel. The post carried with it a professorship on the medical faculty of the university. Here was his chance to settle down and pass on to the young what he had learned.

He announced that his courses were planned to free medicine of its worst errors of the past "[n]ot by following that which those of old taught, but by our own observation of nature, confirmed by extensive practice and long experience."[5]

His program was bound to upset the medical faculty, especially since his fellow professors were already prejudiced against him. They had not been consulted about his appointment. He had presented no credentials, since he had apparently lost his diplomas during his wanderings. His habits, too, were shocking. He refused to wear an academic gown and a doctor's bonnet. He drank heavily and used coarse language. In short, he did not behave like a professor.

The hostility of the faculty he could bear. His hope lay in his students who would carry his message into the future. But they failed to understand him and joined the mounting opposition. In February 1528, Paracelsus left Basel and resumed his wanderings.

Little is known about the final thirteen years of Paracelsus's life. Rumor had it that, as he wandered through Europe, he earned more from wagers that he could outdrink his tavern companions than from the practice of medicine. He carried a massive sword from which he was never parted. The knob on its hilt contained what he called his "stone of immortality." It was generally believed that this "stone" was opium. Was Paracelsus an opium addict as well as a hearty drinker? Nobody knows. But one thing is certain. The stone did not bring him immortality. He died from a wound he received in a tavern brawl in Salzburg at the age of forty-eight.

In England in the sixteenth century the sap of the poppy was regarded as a cure-all for brain disorders, because the poppy head looked like the head of a man. "Aloft in rows large poppy heads were strung"[6] in the apothecary shops of the day.

The Englishman Thomas Sydenham (1624-1689) is generally regarded as one of the founders of clinical medicine. He is credited with saying that without opium the healing art would cease to exist. Also that, of all available remedies, "there is not one that equals opium in its power to moderate the violence of so many maladies, and even to cure some of them."[7]

Sydenham was responsible for the development in 1669 of laudanum in liquid form (tincture of opium) as we know it today. His preparation combined opium and saffron in Canary wine. He wrote: "I do not believe this preparation has more virtues than the solid laudanum of the shops, but it is more convenient to administer."[8]

About the same time, the Netherlander Dr. Franciscus Silvius announced that he would not wish to practice medicine without opium, and the Flemish Jean Baptiste van Helmont (*c.* 1577-1644), a disciple of Paracelsus, became known as "Doctor Opiatus."

More than one account exists as to the early life of Thomas Dover (d. 1742). On the one hand, he is reputed to have been a devoted servant of Thomas Sydenham who left his master to go to sea. On the other, he is said to have been a pupil of Sydenham who practiced medicine in Bristol for twenty-four years and then went to sea. In either case, he wound up as a privateer or gentleman pirate.

On a return to the port of London in 1710 with a captured Spanish frigate and a shipload of treasure, Captain Dover decided he was tired of the sea. He retired and established himself as a London physician, continuing to practice there until his death thirty-two years later. The account that holds him to have been Sydenham's servant has him practicing in London as a free lance or quack. This status seems to be borne out by the fact that the College of Physicians refused to certify him. Dover dismissed its membership as a "clan of most prejudiced gentlemen."[9] However, there is a measure of support for the claim of prior practice in Bristol in a book Dover published before his death. *An Ancient Physician's Legacy to his Country* states on the title page that it is an account of what he had collected in forty-nine years practice.

Whatever his qualifications, Thomas Dover is remembered for his introduction of a medicine for aches and pains that sells to this day. It is known as Dover's powder. It is a combination of opium and ipecac and is effective in small doses.

Dr. Dover himself had no use for small doses. His overdoses

ran to 60-100 grains in contrast with a modern doctor's 5 or less. In fact, eighteenth-century druggists advised patients bringing in a prescription from Dr. Dover to make their wills before taking the powder.

Dover's irresponsible approach went a long way toward destroying the reputation that his master or teacher Sydenham had built up for opium.

Another Englishman, Joshua Ward (1685-1761), started out as a servant, just as Dover may have done. Subsequently he traveled throughout Europe gathering prescriptions written down by monks who doubled as physicians through some centuries of the Middle Ages. Ward returned to England and entered medicine by the back door (as a quack) at the age of forty-eight. He was fortunate enough to become the protégé of King George II.

Ward's secret remedies were powerful. They involved antimony, mercury, opium, arsenic. His Paste, Powder, Pills, Balsam, and Drops continued in use for a century after his death. He unearthed the recipe for Dover's powder from Dover's book and used it effectively, thereby reestablishing its fame. Dover's powder was included in the 1788 edition of the *London Pharmacopoeia*.

One of the earliest and most famous patent medicines was Dr. Bateman's Pectoral Drops. First sold in 1726, it was advertised as a remedy for rheumatism, afflictions of the stone, gravel, agues, and hysterics. It consisted of opium and alcohol seasoned with camphor and anise. Another popular nostrum was Godfrey's Cordial, an elaborate mixture of spices, opium, molasses, and alcohol. A third was Black Drop or "vinegar of opium." It had three times the strength of laudanum and involved the juice of wild crabapples.

Dr. Jacob Le Mort (1650-1718), Professor of Chemistry at the Dutch University of Leyden from 1702 until his death, produced a paregoric (from the Greek word for "soothing") consisting of opium, honey, licorice, benzoic acid, camphor, oil of anise, potassium carbonate, and alcohol. He may well have based

his formula on a seventeenth-century *tinctura anodyna* (an ano-
dyne is also soothing) that involved opium, benzoin, saffron,
alcohol, castor, and salt of tartar.

In the nineteenth century the United States was to develop a
considerable number of unwitting opium addicts among its middle-
aged ladies. They sipped such patent medicines as Mrs. Winslow's
Soothing Syrup and Pierce's Golden Discovery—both generously
laced with opium.

Poppy seed and poppy-seed oil were long used in France in
the preparation of food. But early in the eighteenth century
rumors spread to the effect that poppy seed contained the same
narcotic principles as opium. Reaction was so violent that the
Paris authorities asked the Medical Faculty to investigate. The
Faculty correctly reported that no narcotics were present either
in the seed or the oil. But this did not satisfy the people. Their
clamor forced a 1718 ban on the sale of poppy-seed oil. It was
not lifted until 1773.

One final historical note: The story is told that Napoleon,
returning from his campaign into Egypt and Asia, decided that
his many sick and wounded were so much excess baggage that
were eating up his army's food supplies. He had them fed large
quantities of poppy juice and left them behind to sleep eternally.

SERTUERNER
SEEKS PURE OPIUM

Frederick Wilhelm Sertuerner (1783-1841) was born in the little
German town of Paderborn. At the age of sixteen, he was ap-
prenticed to the royal pharmacist, "Papa" Cramer. He was not
consulted. If he had been, he would have made it plain that he
wanted to be an engineer.

Battle was joined forthwith. Cramer was determined to arouse

Frederick's interest in pharmacy. The young man was firm in his resolve to annoy the boss so much that he would fire him.

Two months went by during which the antagonists did their best and worst. Then one day Cramer announced that the still was not working properly. It would have to be replaced, he said. Not so, retorted the querulous Frederick. He could certainly fix it. The following week the big filter broke down and Frederick fixed it. Then it was the mortar stand. Finally Cramer announced that he needed a better evaporator. Frederick built it. Soon Sertuerner was repairing the apothecary scales and incidentally learning how to weigh drugs. He reorganized the stockroom. When he was done, he was familiar with the Latin names of most of the drugs. Now he was waiting on customers and filling prescriptions. At length he told Cramer that he didn't know how he, Cramer, had managed to get along without him.

Cramer had never given a moment of his life to research but he was craftily leading the would-be engineer into it. How could one measure the amount of benzoic acid in fennel water, he wondered aloud. How much saltpeter was there in sugar beets? Before long Frederick was thinking up projects of his own.

His real opportunity came when the local doctor complained that the opium he bought from Cramer varied in quality. In one case it had made the patient more miserable than his gout did. On the other hand, another batch had rendered a patient unconscious for three days and almost killed her. More recently, ounces of opium had failed to relieve the pain of a little girl whose face, shoulders, and arms had been burned by scalding water.

After the doctor left, Frederick took down the opium jar and rolled some of the powdery gum on the table. He asked Papa Cramer if it was pure.

The old pharmacist was quick to protest the purity of his product. But he called back his words as soon as he had spoken them, admitting that the opium could not be considered pure since it was mixed with oils and salts and possibly some acids.

Young Frederick voiced the opinion that the oils and salts in no way contributed to the painkilling properties of opium. On the other hand, their presence could account for the fact that the opium provided to the local doctor was sometimes too strong and sometimes too weak.

He proposed that they go to work to extract *pure* opium.

Cramer would personally have none of it, but he had laid the groundwork well. Sertuerner was determined.

He completed his four-year apprenticeship. He passed his pharmacist's examination and returned to Cramer as employee. Night after night found young Sertuerner trying test after test.

He preferred playing hunches to attacking the problem systematically. One night he got the idea of neutralizing the acid solution with alkaline ammonia. The solution became hot when he poured the ammonia in. As it cooled, a batch of crystals appeared in what had been water-clear liquid. It was 1803. Sertuerner was then twenty.

The crystals were gray; opium was brown. Perhaps the crystals were the something that stopped pain. It turned out that they were not. What Sertuerner did not then know was that, contained in the gray crystals, were the white crystals of another substance that would one day revolutionize the practice of medicine.

However, after further months of testing, Sertuerner began to *suspect* the presence of an additional substance. He was forced to the conclusion that it was an alkali, present in the crude opium and unrelated to the alkaline ammonia. He found this hard to accept. According to his textbooks, plants did not contain alkalies. Finally he decided that his textbooks were wrong.

Working surreptitiously, he tried out his alkaloid—the designation by which morphine, atropine, quinine, strychnine, and other plant derivatives would later be known—on rats, mice, cats, and dogs. The crystals, while odorless, were quite bitter, but he was able to disguise the taste with sugar syrup.

His crystals produced sleep, but would his test animals wake?

He gave his first dog five grains. It slept for two days and then died. The next dog died in a coma following a dose of two and a half grams. Gradually he worked down to the right dosage. At length he could put animals to sleep with reasonable assurance that they would wake again.

MORPHINE

When Sertuerner first precipitated the gray crystals in 1803, he submitted a report of his discovery to Professor Trommsdorff of the University of Erfurt. Trommsdorff condemned the report as "juvenile prattle," but he nonetheless published it in his journal. Now Sertuerner wrote to Trommsdorff again.

"I have been fortunate enough to find in opium still another substance which has been unknown until now. . . . It is neither earth, gluten or resin, nor the compound I found last year, but an entirely individual one. The substance is the specific narcotic element of opium . . . the *Principium somniferum.*"[10]

Trommsdorff also published this report but damned it with faint praise: "The experiments contain many interesting suggestions, but we can by no means consider that the work on opium is concluded. . . . *There have been so many works on opium.* . . ."[11]

The young pharmacist was bitter. He had solved the mystery of opium, without training, help, or adequate equipment, only to be slapped down by the great Trommsdorff. Frederick Wilhelm Sertuerner swore that he would never touch opium again.

In 1806, at the age of twenty-three, he left Cramer and moved to the nearby town of Einbeck in South Hanover. He took a job as assistant at the city pharmacy. For a time he limited himself to the discouraging task of dispensing drugs, but eventually he drifted back into research. He did good work on caustic soda and caustic potash and in galvanism. However, he could not get his results published.

"It's a conspiracy . . . against all Germans," he complained. "We can't get recognition, even in our own country."[12]

He abandoned drugs in disgust and turned successfully to the manufacture of munitions.

His return to opium was accidental. He awoke one night with a raging toothache. Looking for something to quiet it, he came upon a supply of his *Principium somniferum* that he had not thrown out when he left the drug field. He combined a small quantity with sugar syrup and gulped down the mixture. It had worked with dogs, he told himself, why not man? He figured to put himself to sleep for half an hour. He woke eight hours later. The pain was entirely gone. By a happy chance he had proved to his own satisfaction that his white crystals might safely be taken by human beings.

But one case, with himself as guinea pig and no witnesses, would certainly not satisfy skeptical scientists and doctors.

He got hold of three young men of the town who boasted that they were afraid of nothing. They agreed to join him in taking the "magic crystals."

The experiment did not go as smoothly as he might have hoped, but at least all four of them survived their sleep. Sertuerner named his crystals *morphine* after Morpheus, the Greek god of dreams.

Sertuerner wrote a report on his latest experiments and findings and submitted it to Ludwig Gilbert of Leipzig. Gilbert published it in 1815, but he added that he did so "against our better judgement [as] highly unscientific and unchemical; if there is such a thing as Sertuerner's 'morphine,' we chemists have much new to learn. . . ."[13]

Here was the condemning Trommsdorff all over again. Sertuerner was in despair. Fortunately the article was read by the celebrated French chemist Joseph Louis Gay-Lussac. He wrote that Sertuerner's "discovery of his alkaline base, morphine, appears to us to be of the greatest importance. . . ." Gay-Lussac went even further. He instructed his students at the Sorbonne: "Read what

M. Sertuerner has discovered in opium. Read about his morphine. See what this scientist has accomplished without help, without funds, without training, with the most simple apparatus. Gentlemen, M. Sertuerner can teach us all how to perform experiments!"[14]

Sertuerner became famous overnight. Then others tried to climb on the bandwagon, each with the claim that he had discovered morphine first.

It was in 1804 that Sertuerner announced his isolation of the white crystals that he would later name morphine. About the time that he precipitated his ineffectual gray crystals a year earlier, a Parisian chemist, Charles Derosne, thought he had discovered the active principle of opium. He described his findings in the *Annales de Chimie* for February 1804, naming his product *narcotine*. Narcotine turned out to be merely one of the alkaloids of opium, and it was misnamed. It possessed absolutely no narcotic properties. This in itself would discredit any claim on Derosne's part to be the discoverer of morphine.

The claim of another French chemist, Sequin by name, had greater surface validity. In December 1804, Sequin described a process for producing an alkaloid of opium. He was obviously on the track of morphine. His paper on the subject was not published until ten years later, but its publication was nonetheless a year ahead of Sertuerner's paper announcing morphine. However, Sequin's claim to have been the discoverer of morphine is somewhat diluted by the fact that, even in 1814, he did not recognize the pharmacological significance of his discovery.

This circumstance of rival discoverers arriving at their conclusions about the same time is not unusual in scientific research. A famous recent case involved the structure of deoxyribonucleic acid (DNA), described by the American molecular biologist James D. Watson and the British biologist Francis H. C. Crick in 1953 as the *double helix*. Late the previous year, Watson and Crick thought they had been beaten to the post by Linus Pauling of California Institute of Technology, but the latter scientist had fallen into a chemical error. In the summer of 1955, Watson was to write ". . . [In 1951] DNA was still a mystery, up for grabs. . . . Chiefly it was a matter of five people: Maurice Wilkins, Rosalind Franklin, Linus Pauling, Francis Crick, and me."[15]

In the morphine case, Sertuerner certainly deserved the credit finally accorded him. He had spent many years pursuing the active principle of opium and had recognized it and confirmed it when he at last succeeded.

But the infighting after his announcement was made disgusted him. The recognition that should have been his earlier did not come until 1831. Then the French Institute awarded him a prize of 2000 francs for having opened the way to important medical discoveries by his isolation of morphine and his exposition of its character.

By then he had retired and married and was raising a family. He lived another ten years after this belated recognition. But his final year was passed in terrible pain.

Ironically, the man who had turned treacherous opium into reliable morphine could not benefit from his discovery. He was too weak to swallow morphine and, in 1841, the hypodermic needle had not yet been perfected.

DEVELOPMENT OF
THE HYPODERMIC NEEDLE

In the first century A.D. Hero of Alexandria devised a "machine" consisting of a cylinder and a tight-fitting plunger that squirted out liquid. Early in the seventeenth century, England's William Harvey (1578-1657) established that the blood circulates throughout the body, leaving the heart through the arteries and returning through the veins. By the middle of the nineteenth century, it was time to make a combined use of Hero's machine and Harvey's discovery.

A major problem attached to the use of opium or Sertuerner's morphine. To be effective as a painkiller, the drug had to reach the brain, the seat of the central nervous system, as quickly as possible. Opium introduced into the stomach by mouth moved slowly and not always in the right direction. Opium introduced by means of a rectal enema proved no more effective. Attempts were made to introduce it through the lungs by the smoking of opium, but much of the active principle was dissipated in the process of combustion. The bloodstream was the obvious route to the brain. How could morphine be introduced into the bloodstream? Obviously a small version of Hero's syringe was needed.

A number of doctors went to work on its development. In 1845 Francis Rynd of Dublin produced a primitive device. Charles-Gabriel Provas in France followed suit in 1851. But it was left to the Scotsman Alexander Wood (1817-1884) to perfect the hypodermic needle in 1853. Five years later two Americans, Fordyce Barker and George Thompson, introduced injected morphine into medical practice—just in time for the Civil War.

Dr. Wood lived to regret his invention. His wife was the first person to acquire the morphine-by-needle habit. She died from an overdose of morphine. Doctors chose to ignore this tragedy. Mrs. Wood's death was an unfortunate exception. They could readily imagine addiction arising from morphine taken by mouth because of different body reactions and tolerances. But they were satisfied that there could be no danger from injected morphine which could be closely controlled.

How wrong they were was dramatically demonstrated by the number of morphine "addicts" that returned from the Civil War.

A score of opium alkaloids exist, but only three are in common, if strictly limited, use today. They are morphine, codeine, and papaverine. Morphine and codeine act on the central nervous system. Morphine is a painkiller. Codeine is mainly used to control coughing. It is not as habit-forming as morphine. Papaverine has little effect on the nervous system but effectively relaxes certain muscles. Papaverine is not generally regarded as habit forming.

OPIUM ADDICTION
BROUGHT TO CHINA

In Persia and China the dried sap of the plant of joy was smoked; in India opium was eaten. But until 250 years ago the amount consumed for nonmedical purposes was minimal. In fact, while opium eating in India began a thousand years ago, the Indians are said to have thought of it strictly as a medicine—the more so because it had a nasty taste.

Poppies had been grown in Chinese gardens for their decorative value since the Sung dynasty (tenth-thirteenth centuries A.D.) and Chinese physicians had long regarded opium as a highly important drug. But, prior to the eighteenth century, the use of opium as a pleasure drug had not been widespread.

In 1644 the Emperor Tsung Cheng had prohibited tobacco smoking, a habit introduced into China by Dutch and Portuguese sailors. The Chinese took up opium smoking instead. Within a hundred years this new habit had become enough of a problem to require the issuing, in 1729, of a severe edict against opium. The keepers of opium shops were to be strangled. Their assistants were to receive a hundred lashes with a bamboo cane followed by three months in prison and banishment thereafter to at least a thousand miles from their former homes. Boatmen, soldiers, police, custom officials, and neighbors who traded in or shut their eyes to the passage of opium would be similarly punished. The addicts themselves were left undisturbed.

The 1729 edict proved largely ineffective. The British East India Company began flooding Chinese seaports with cheap India-grown opium. (Downtrodden coolies were quick to accept this easy escape from reality.) Once the Chinese were hooked, the price was eased upward, but it made no difference. Shipments rose from 1,000 chests of opium annually in 1767 to 4,244 in 1820 and 78,354 in 1854. Opium was now big business.

Chinese dealers jumped into the market. Soon poppies cultivated in China produced more than enough opium to meet local demands with some left over for export. Imports of opium were barred. But the English merchants were not to be outdone. Claiming that they were only giving the Chinese what they wanted, they bribed officials and engaged in smuggling. Their fast boats easily outsailed the Chinese war junks. Addicts were created to smoke away the surplus supplies. Opium became a more acceptable medium of exchange than silver dollars.

As a retaliatory step, Chinese authorities required all foreigners to surrender any opium in their possession and sign bonds for their future collective good conduct. The British responded in 1839 with a declaration of war. This Opium War ended in 1842 in a decisive British victory. The concluding Treaty of Nanking not only required China to pay British opium traders for all the losses they had sustained but also declared opium an article of commerce. Opium was in China to stay.

ADDICTION AMONG BRITISH AND AMERICAN WRITERS

Until a generation ago, most people thought that all opium eaters and smokers were skid-row bums, underfed Chinese coolies, or Indian untouchables. This was never true. The white man may have forced the habit on the "heathen Chinee," but he was more than repaid by the number of his talented writers (to select a single group) who became addicted to opium.

The English poet George Crabbe started the opium habit when he was working as an apothecary and had not abandoned it prior to his death at age seventy-seven.

Walter Scott is best known to most of us for his adventurous historical novels. However, his mystical *The Bride of Lammermoor* is usually regarded as his most beautiful work. The book is so superior to anything else he wrote that it has even been suggested that it was written by someone else. The truth seems to be that he wrote it during a series of opium trips. He started taking the drug to relieve him of the pain of gallstone spasms.

Samuel Taylor Coleridge began taking Kendal's Black Drop (a camphorated solution of opium) at the age of nineteen to combat arthritic pain and swelling resulting from rheumatic fever. He continued taking opium during the remaining forty-three years of his life. He would drink as much as half a pint of laudanum at a time. He said that he took opium "as a means of escape from pain that coiled around my mental powers as a serpent around the body and wings of an eagle."[16] He spent his last days in the company of a sympathetic physician whose chief service was to ration his doses of laudanum.

Thomas De Quincey began taking enormous quantities of opium at age twenty-seven. He broke the habit at thirty-seven and lived to be seventy-four. Unfortunately, his *Confessions of an English Opium-Eater* led many thousands to addiction.

Roughly 130 years ago Edgar Allan Poe, who left behind him some exceptional poetry and prose, was stumbling about the streets of Philadelphia, drunk and drugged with opium. Doors were slammed in his face when he applied for the humblest of jobs.

Wilkie Collins, celebrated as the author of *The Moonstone,* was a morphine addict.

Francis Thompson became addicted to morphine at the age

of nineteen. He took it to escape the frustrations and cruelties of life. His opium dreams are well reflected in such poems as the mystical *The Hound of Heaven*. He ended his life in poverty, sponging on women, as Poe also did.

INTRODUCTION
OF HEROIN

In 1898, Professor Heinrich Dreser of the German Bayer Works announced that he had created a drug that not only did the work of morphine but was safe and nonaddictive.

He named his safe pain-killing drug *heroin*.

How tragically wrong his evaluation turned out to be!

Almost three-quarters of a century later, in 1970, Milt Freudenheim could write in the *Chicago Daily News:* "The French Corsican underworld's heroin factories, hidden around Marseilles, have shifted to around-the-clock production to meet soaring demand from the United States.

"As heroin addiction among young Americans spreads to university campuses and middle-class suburbs, the gangster supply system stretching from Turkey via Marseilles to New York is racing to keep up."[17]

Heroin, a hydrochloride derivative of morphine, is one of the *easiest* drugs to become addicted to. On the other hand, it has been called ". . . the hardest of drugs . . . the toughest of monkeys for anyone to get off his back."[18]

Heroin never became highly regarded in medicine and has in fact been outlawed by the United Nations Technical Committee. Consequently, it is produced *solely* for illegal sale to addicts.

Attempts to restrict the production (and illegal sale) of opium were begun in 1906. The British House of Commons carried a motion stating "That this House reaffirms its conviction that the

Indo-Chinese opium trade is morally indefensible, and requests His Majesty's Government to take such steps as may be necessary for bringing about its speedy close."[19] The Secretary of State for India retorted that the first step must be taken by China, since she was a producing country. China reacted by initiating legislation aimed at ending all opium production within ten years. In 1908, Britain agreed to reduce Indian exports in proportion to China's reductions in cultivation. So much for one-quarter of the world.

President Theodore Roosevelt was responsible for calling the first international conference on opium. Annexation of the Philippines in 1898 had introduced the United States to the world-wide implications of the opium trade. The victor of San Juan Hill was again ready to charge.

However, it was 1909 before the International Opium Commission met in Shanghai. Austria-Hungary, the British Empire, China, France, Germany, Italy, Japan, the Netherlands, Persia, Portugal, Russia, Siam, and the United States were represented. Turkey, a producer, was invited but declined the invitation. The assembled representatives resolved that "the use of opium and its alkaloids for nonmedical purposes was evil, was spreading, and is to be restrained. . . ."[20] It was a beginning.

In 1912 The Hague International Opium Convention was held at the seat of the Permanent Court of International Justice. More might have been achieved than actually resulted if World War I had not followed close on its heels. Subsequently the League of Nations took up the cause but with little concrete success.

World War II reestablished the medical value of opium. In the front lines with the troops or under the blitz in cities like London, opium (or morphine) was unequaled as a soother of pain. Without it, many who survived might not have.

Today the production of opium-morphine-heroin is technically controlled by the World Health Organization. But opium far in excess of medical needs is still produced. There is widespread addiction in India, Iran, and in and around Yugoslavia. There is no reason to suppose that the Communists have driven the habit out of China.

And then there is the United States, which has long had heroin addiction. Until recent years, however, Americans consoled themselves with the thought that it was an affliction of the criminal, the self-indulgent, and the derelict. Now there is a heroin "epidemic" among the young. In New York City in 1969 one-quarter of the deaths from heroin overdose involved teenagers. It was estimated that by mid-1970 there would be 100,000 young addicts in New York City, perhaps a quarter of a million countrywide. This is quite an introduction to the soaring seventies.

In the 1950s and early 1960s, the game was "chicken"—two stripped-down "buggies" in a head-on crash path and thumbs down on the one who chickened out first. Chicken was then the means of gaining the respect of one's peers. Now it is shooting the most dangerous drug that can be found. The price has gone up in terms of an entrapment that can only lead to a losing financial battle and moral deterioration. In the game of chicken, you chickened out and lived or held your course and maybe died. It was all very sudden. With heroin, you are trapped before you have enough information to make a choice, and only the lucky ones die.

There will be a solution because there must be. Perhaps a strict international agreement limiting opium poppy production to medical needs may yet be worked out and ratified. Turkey is a major producer. Her neighbor, Iran, quit growing opium poppies in 1956. The Turkish government cut its planted acreage in half in 1967-69. There is now a U.S.-backed move to help Turkey face the economic problem involved in giving up opium production altogether. If the world supply of heroin can be eliminated, it will be impossible to make the scene.

This can only be for the best. As J. M. Scott has written, ". . . those who have suffered a painful operation and have been given heroin or one of its sisters know the mood that we associate with heaven. Those who take it for other reasons commit the unforgivable sin against themselves."[21]

The pretty, fragile white poppy, without thorn or sting, has been aptly described, also by Scott, as "the plant of good and evil."[22]

Opium was the earliest known painkiller, but it was not the only analgesic to be derived from plant life.

The leaf of the South American coca plant was first used to deaden pain about eight hundred years ago. Unfortunately, it revealed the good and evil qualities already seen in opium.

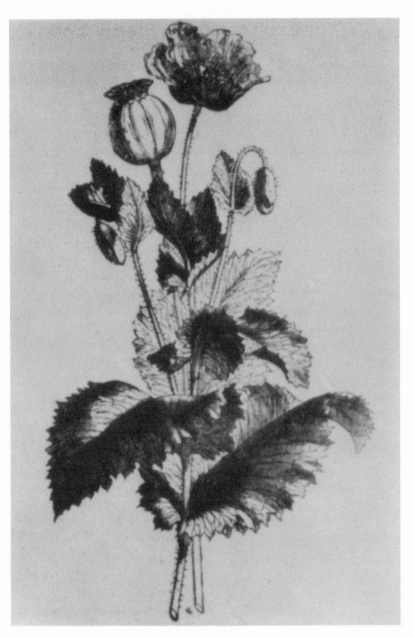

1. Opium poppy

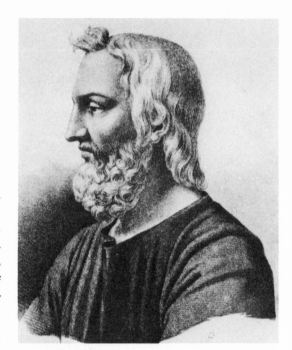

*2. Pedanios
Dioskorides, who
described over
1,000 years ago the
method still used to
collect the sap of
the poppy*

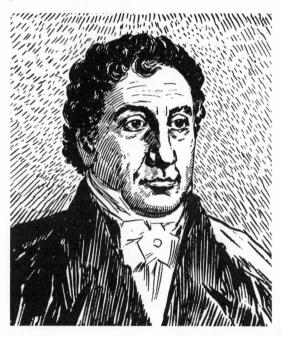

*3. Frederick Wilhelm
Sertuerner, who
isolated morphine*

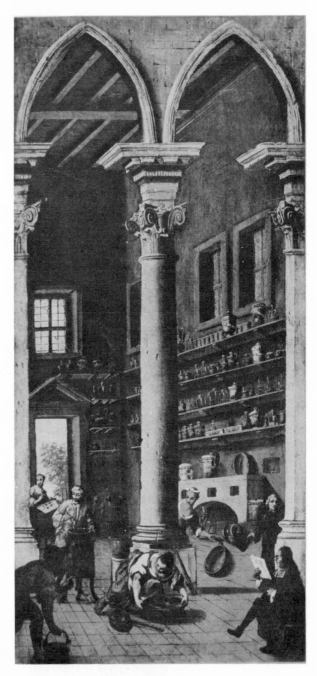

4. Seventeenth-century Italian pharmacy

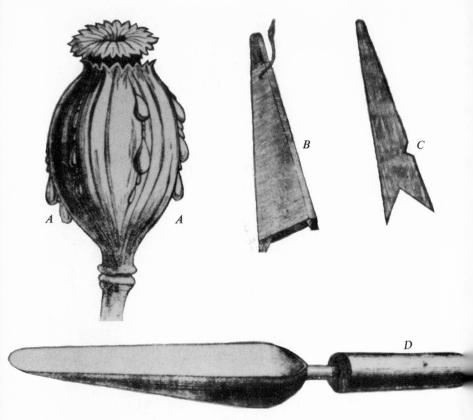

5. Tools used in the collection of opium
  A. Crude opium exuding from the green poppy head
  B. Knife with four double-pointed blades for scratching the green capsule
  C. One of the blades of the knife
  D. Iron spoon for collecting the drops of opium

  The poppy head and the knife are actual size; the spoon is half actual size

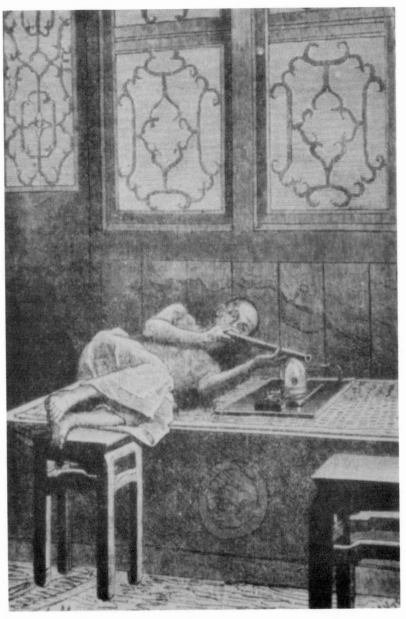

6. *Opium smoker*

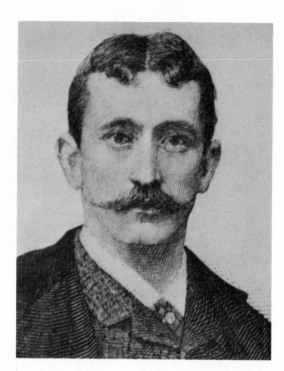

7. Carl Koller, who
initiated local
anesthesia for the eye

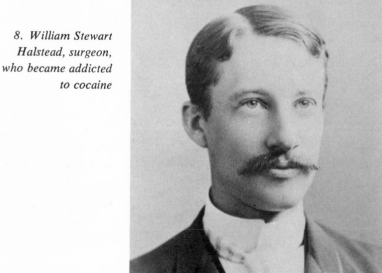

8. William Stewart
Halstead, surgeon,
who became addicted
to cocaine

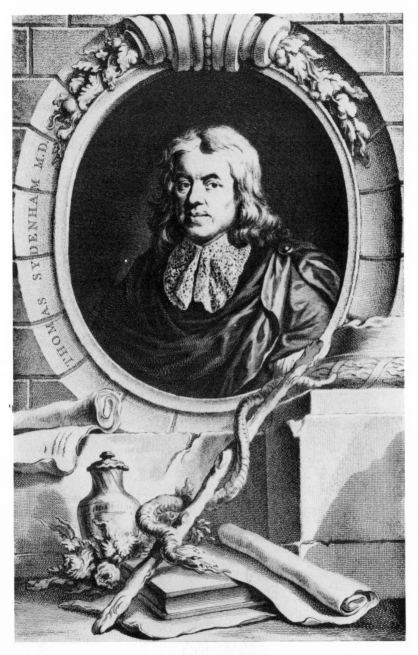

9. *Thomas Sydenham, who reversed himself in
regard to Peruvian bark*

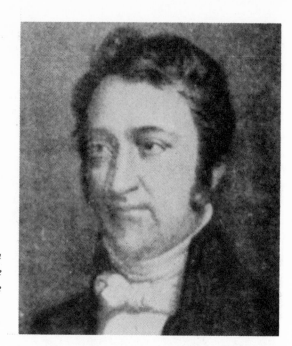

*10. Pierre Joseph
Pelletier, one of the
developers of quinine*

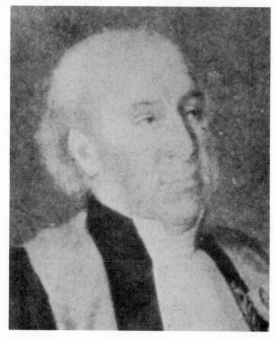

*11. Joseph Bienaimé
Caventou, who
worked with Pelletier*

12. Statue of Pelletier and Caventou on the Boulevard St. Michel in Paris, erected in 1900 by popular subscription

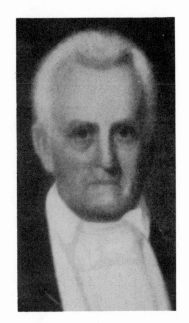

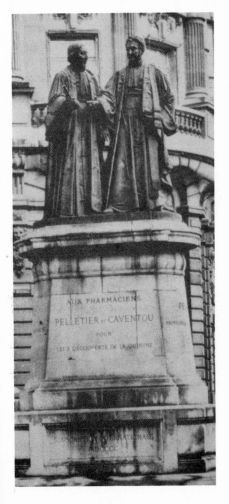

13. John Sappington, midwest physician, whose fever pills checked malaria in the Mississippi Valley. From a portrait by George Caleb Bingham

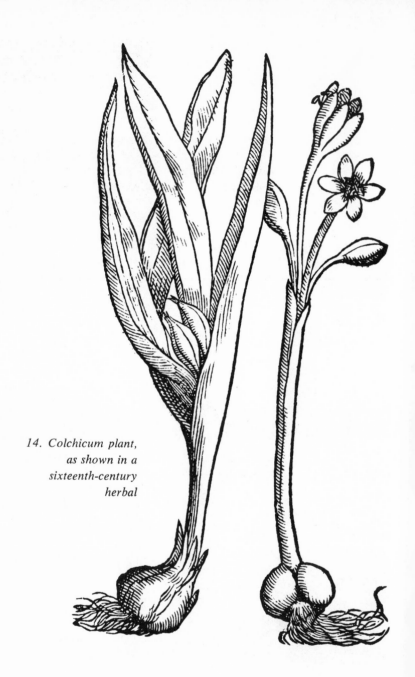

*14. Colchicum plant,
as shown in a
sixteenth-century
herbal*

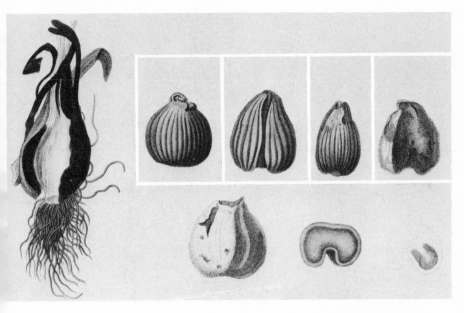

15. *Corms of the autumn crocus*

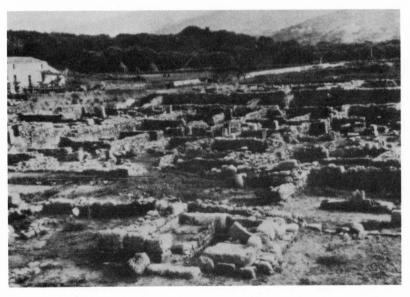

16. *Ruins of the Salerno medical school, the first in Europe, where colchicum therapy was taught as early as the eleventh century*

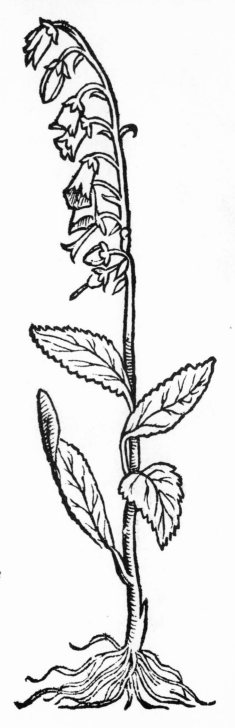

17. Foxglove plant

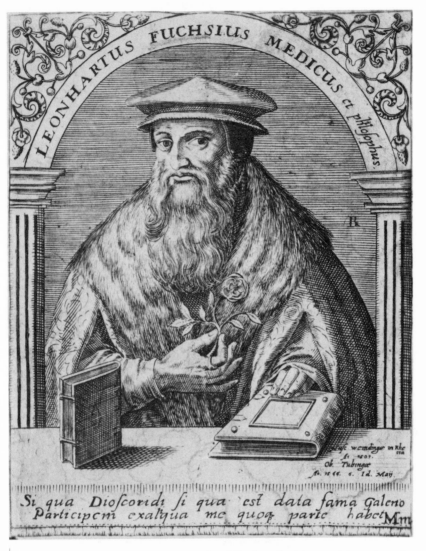

LEONHARTUS FUCHSIUS MEDICUS et philosophus.

Si qua Dioscoridi si qua est data fama Galeno
Participem exalqua me quoq parte habet

18. *Leonhard Fuchs, physician and botanist, who
included foxglove in his history of plants*

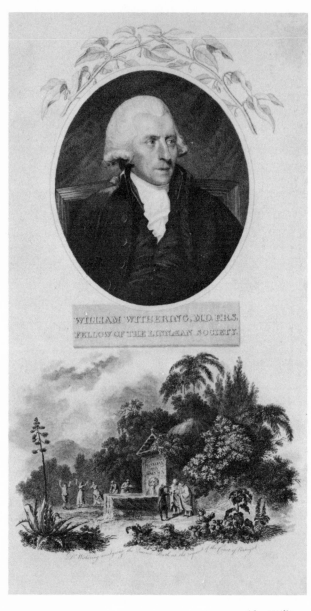

WILLIAM WITHERING, M.D. F.R.S.
FELLOW OF THE LINNEAN SOCIETY.

19. William
Withering, who
turned an old wives'
tale into a medical
reality

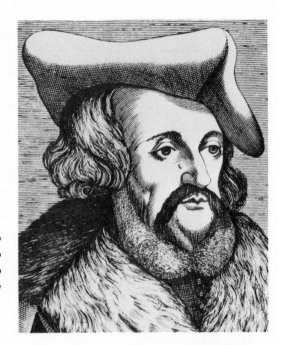

*20. Girolamo
Fracastoro, who
pointed the way to
bacteriology*

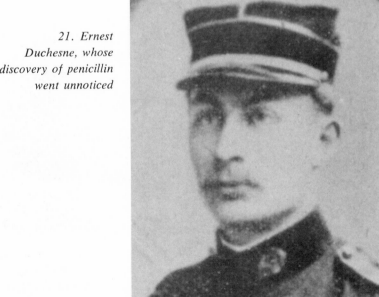

*21. Ernest
Duchesne, whose
discovery of penicillin
went unnoticed*

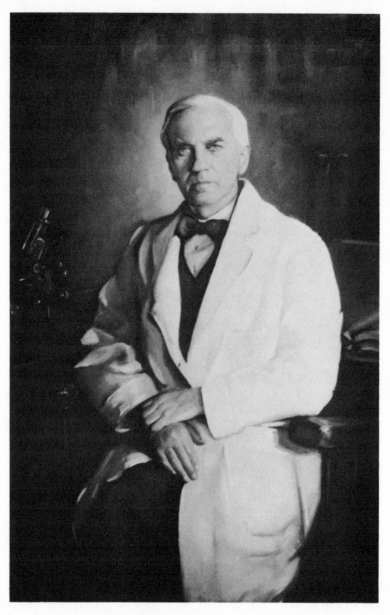

22. *Alexander Fleming, whose isolation of penicillin gained him a Nobel prize*

Two

The Divine Plant
of the Incas
⁓ Cocaine

THE HERB
CALLED COCA

"In certain valleys, among the mountains [of Peru], there grows a certain herb called Coca, which the Indians do esteem more than gold or silver. . . . The virtue of this herb found by experience is that any man having these leaves hath never hunger or thirst. . . ."[1] This was part of the report of the Spanish explorer Augostín de Zárate, made on his return to Spain from Peru in 1555. He would never have believed what he had seen if he had simply been told about it. But he had witnessed it with his own eyes.

The thin mountain air in the high Andes is freezing cold. Nevertheless de Zárate saw men toiling naked in the gold and silver mines that had been worked by the Purics long before the Spanish conquest of South America. But that was not all. The Indian workers brought out of the mines for de Zárate's inspection had been steadily at work for thirty-six hours, without sleep, food, or water.

The naked Indians paid little attention to their audience. They crouched on their heels in a circle around two pouches on the ground. Each native took a handful of dry, crumbly leaves from one pouch and dipped them in powdered lime from the other. Then he rolled the leaves and lime into a ball, put the ball in his mouth, and chewed on it happily.

De Zárate's guide explained that this practice had come down from the Incas and that it was believed that chewing the leaves enabled men to go without food, water, and sleep, to keep warm while others froze, and to remain fresh after hours of work. The coca leaf even made brave men out of cowards.

31

When he had finished, de Zárate spoke slowly. "I believe you. I believe every word," he said. "And yet when I tell all this in Spain—will they believe me?"[2]

He was right. For two hundred years *Erythroxylon coca* would remain a botanical curiosity with medical pretensions that most physicians laughed at.

THE SPANISH
CONQUEST

The Peruvian Indian had not always been allowed to enjoy the pleasant stimulation of coca chewing.

Before the Spanish conquest, the Inca nation at the height of its power had boasted a population in excess of ten million. Spread over what is now Peru, Bolivia, Ecuador, and parts of Chile and Colombia, this people was segregated into three rigidly distinct classes. At the apex was a small, exclusive group consisting of the reigning Inca, his family, and related aristocrats. They were known as the Incas. Then came the Curacas or provincial nobles. The Curacas were largely the chieftains and officials of subjugated nations and tribes. Finally, the Purics or commoners numbered almost ten million. Thus the Incas in particular, and the Curacas to only slightly a lesser degree, were a privileged few.

Among the privileges these few enjoyed was the right to chew the coca leaf. Actually, this right was regarded as the highest reward the reigning Inca could confer. It was prized far above the richest presents of silver or gold. Consequently, it was a rare thing for the Puric to get to chew the coca leaf. When he did, it was on a special occasion, certainly not as a regular thing.

But all this was changed with the conquest of Peru by the Spaniard Francisco Pizarro at the start of the sixteenth century. The highly organized governmental structure of the Inca empire quickly arrived at a point of collapse. Many of the Incas and Curacas were executed. Those who escaped death disappeared. The Purics survived because of their sheer numbers.

The Spanish conquerors needed these natives to work the gold and silver mines. It did not take them long to recognize that nothing could subdue the Purics more effectively than the coca leaf and the craving for it that followed its use. But subjugation was not all. The Indian on coca could be counted on to work longer and harder and to consume less food.

The Spaniards also needed Indians to run through the mountains as messengers. Obviously, the less messengers must carry, including food and blankets, the faster time they could make. There are accounts of Bolivian Indians known as *andadores* (swift travelers) who covered sixty or seventy miles a day, through mountain passes, for several successive days, sustained only by coca and a little powdered corn. During the Bolivian war of independence, an armed battalion of Indian infantry made forced marches of sixty miles a day, while another battalion under General Valdes covered 108 miles in three days, with nothing to sustain them but coca leaves. But the prize for speed and endurance must go to the Indian who covered 250 miles between La Paz and Taena in four days, rested one day, and returned in five days over a mountain 13,000 feet high.

The Purics, who had never had anything, readily accepted from their new masters "the highest reward the Inca could give."[3] Coca chewing helped them to endure, to forget, and to escape their misery.

Writing three hundred years later, in 1847, William H. Prescott had this to say of the coca tree and its leaves: "This is a shrub that grows to the height of a man. The leaves when gathered are dried in the sun and being mixed with a little lime form a preparation for chewing much like the betel nut of the East. With a small quantity of this coca in his pouch and a handful of roasted maise, the Peruvian Indian of our time performs his wearisome journeys

day after day without fatigue, or at least without complaint. . . .
Under the Incas it is said to have been exclusively reserved for
the noble orders. If so, the people gained one luxury by the conquest."[4]

But this "gain" was of doubtful value to the enslaved Purics.
Their number was reduced from almost ten million to less than
two million in the fifty years following the conquest. To make
matters worse, the occupations the survivors might follow were
restricted. They might work in the silver and gold mines, on the
coca plantations, and in the mills that produced coarse cloth.
They could be household servants. It was to be expected that they
were not allowed to hold public office. But when one realizes that
they were not permitted to trade in the streets, let alone operate
a shop, it becomes obvious how limited their opportunity to
advance really was. Furthermore, heavy taxation kept them constantly in debt. Ironically, part of these taxes had to be paid in
coca leaves, which their masters were finding a very profitable
item of trade.

MARIANI
WINE

In 1735, a French expedition set out for Quito, Ecuador. Its purpose was to measure an arc of the meridian and thereby verify the
shape of the earth. A member of the expedition was a botanist-
physician named Joseph de Jussieu (1704-1779). When the expedition returned to France seven years later, de Jussieu moved on
to Peru. He stayed there for thirty years, collecting plants in the
deep forest, the high mountain passes, and the muddy swamps.

He was among the first to classify *Erythroxylon coca.* He sent
specimens of the plant to Paris where they are preserved to this
day in the Herbarium of the Museum of Natural History.

As the years went by, an increasing number of geographers, naturalists, botanists, and zoologists from France, England, Germany, Italy, and North America journeyed to South America. One of their purposes was to study the plant life.

Because of the similarity in names, many of them confused the coca tree with the cacao trees of Brazil, from which we get cocoa and chocolate. But once the difference was made clear, they were quite uncritical in their acceptance of the stories told of coca. These went beyond the generally recognized claims that coca diminished the need for food, water, and sleep, neutralized the effects of heat and cold, and made brave men out of cowards. It was suggested that coca cured sickness and quieted mental and emotional distress.

However, two Germans, Edouard Poeppig and J. J. von Tschudi, had their doubts not only about the medicinal value of the coca leaf but also about the widely accepted advantages claimed for it. They pointed to the yellowish skin, the pale lips, the greenish, broken-down teeth, the bad breath, the unseeing eyes, the unsteady walk, the general apathy, and the incurable insomnia of the coca-chewers. They noted that white men who started chewing coca could not stop.

But other scientists were not to be turned aside. They first accused Poeppig and von Tschudi of confusing coca with opium. When they could not make this stick, they allowed that the Germans might have seen a few cases of addiction, but these obviously were the exceptions that prove the rule.

The enthusiasm was carried back to Paris where Dr. Angelo Mariani, a young Corsican, saw visions of a tonic that would overcome hunger, fatigue, and cold. He tried to raise coca trees in his garden. When they failed to grow, he imported pound upon pound of coca leaves from South America. Soon he was flooding the market with Mariani wine, Mariani elixir, Mariani lozenges, Mariani tea, and Mariani pastilles. Pope Leo XIII and the French composers Charles Gounod and Jules Massenet were among his satisfied customers.

Doctors were as loud as anyone in singing the praises of the Mariani products. Dr. Charles Fauvel of Paris reported that Mariani wine had restored the voices of opera singers who would not otherwise have been able to perform. The Abbé Pullez confessed that he took coca two days in advance when he was scheduled to preach a long sermon. He found that it increased the quality and volume of his voice. The as yet unrecognized anesthetic effect of coca was doing wonders.

Ranging farther afield, Dr. Marius Odin told of a young woman suffering from insomnia and night problems. Mariani wine cured the headaches, dizziness, fatness, depression, and general weakness and debility that were the causes of her night problems. Before long coca had earned a firm reputation of relieving such common distresses as stomachache, indigestion, headache, dizziness, sore throat, seasickness, constipation, paleness, irritability, and insomnia. In addition it was regarded as a cure for anemia, nervous exhaustion, diabetes, Bright's disease, gout, rheumatism, heart disease, tuberculosis, malaria, goiter, convulsions, and syphilis. It was reported from Boston that coca dissipates "the blues"; New York regarded it as an excellent general tonic; Columbus, Ohio, viewed it as "a tonic in dyspepsia and nervous prostration"; London found it "a valuable stimulant."[5]

But there were some who were not ready to jump on the bandwagon. Thomás Moreno y Maiz, a former chief surgeon of the Peruvian army, even questioned the effectiveness of coca as a hunger preventive and a reducer of the need for food. He separated an equal number of fat, healthy rats in two cages. One group was left to starve. The other was put on a diet of coca leaves. The rats fed on coca died sooner than the rats fed nothing.

Moreno y Maiz had set his foot on a path which would, a few years later, lead him close, though because of his caution not close enough, to the truth about coca leaves.

Chewing them did in effect eliminate the need for food, water, and sleep; it did overcome fatigue; it did protect against extremes of temperature; it did relieve the pain of sickness, and so on. But this was thanks to an anesthetizing quality, not to some special virtue that coca alone possessed. In short, it did not eliminate the ordinary needs of man; it merely masked them.

NIEMANN
ISOLATES COCAINE

In 1806, José Hipolito de Unanue, who had described many Peruvian diseases and plants, came close to discovering the active principle of coca leaves. By 1850, a Dr. Weddell had undertaken numerous experiments directed toward determining their composition. But it remained for Albert Niemann (d. 1877), a German chemist, to announce in 1860 that he had successfully isolated from coca leaves an alkaloid to which he gave the name *cocaine*.

Niemann's report on cocaine included a subsidiary announcement that did not receive the attention it deserved. He stated that he had put some cocaine in his mouth and had been amazed to discover that his tongue went numb, that he could taste nothing, and that he could not distinguish between hot and cold.

Nineteenth-century physicians paid little attention to reports in chemical and other not strictly medical journals, if they read them at all. Niemann's discoveries went largely unnoticed. The same was true in 1862 when a Viennese pharmacist, Dr. Schroff, reported in another neglected journal that cocaine had produced numbness in his tongue, mouth, and throat. Then a Russian physiologist wrote a paper on the insensitivity produced in animals by applications and injections of cocaine solutions, and a Peruvian doctor found that cocaine compresses relieved painful bruises. But no one appeared to regard these findings as important.

In 1868, Moreno y Maiz, whose earlier experiments have already been discussed, injected a cocaine solution into the hind legs of bullfrogs. The frogs did not jump when he jabbed sharp needles into the injected legs. But they *moved* when he stuck the needles into the motor nerves. This led him to a hesitant conclusion that cocaine completely eliminated local sensation without interfering with the power to move. "The local action of this substance is very marked," he wrote. "Could one utilize cocaine as a local anesthetic? One cannot make a decision on the basis of such a limited number of experiments; it must be decided by the future. . . ."[6]

Moreno y Maiz was professionally overcautious. Had he not been, he might have enjoyed the fame that would come to Carl Koller sixteen years later.

He was not alone in missing the boat. There was also the German eye specialist who described the numbness produced by cocaine to a group of ear-eye-nose-and-throat specialists as a great joke.

But as Francis Darwin has said: "In science the credit goes to the man who convinces the world, not to the man to whom the idea first occurs."[7]

FREUD UNDERTAKES
A PROJECT

In the summer of 1884, two young men sat in the office of Dr. Josef Breuer (1842-1925) at the General Hospital in Vienna. Sigmund Freud (1856-1939) at twenty-eight had not yet embarked on his career in psychoanalysis. Carl Koller (1857-1944) was slightly younger. They were discussing one of Dr. Freud's patients. Dr. Breuer pointed out that he seemed to have become addicted to cocaine.

Freud rejected the suggestion. He was prepared to admit that his patient might have been poisoned by cocaine—that he might have given him too much of the drug. But he was quite positive that he could not have become addicted. After all, it had been clearly demonstrated in America that cocaine is not addicting.

Dr. Breuer asked what Freud meant when he spoke of clear demonstration in America. Freud cited two reports published there four years earlier.

The first was by a Rockford, Illinois, physician who announced a new cure for the opium habit. He had found that slaves to the juice of the poppy could successfully substitute a fluid extract of coca for morphine. Patients so treated had no difficulty in subsequently giving up coca. Then a Dr. E. C. Bentley of Valley Oak, Kentucky, not only confirmed his colleague's findings but went on to state that coca cured alcoholism in addition to the opium habit. Freud did not hesitate to press his opinion that in a few years morphine addiction would be completely wiped out.

Breuer said he hoped Freud was right but insisted that the case under consideration lent little encouragement to the theory. The patient in point was a physician who had become addicted to morphine after having his left thumb amputated. When an attempt was made to withdraw the morphine, the patient suffered so much that Freud had substituted cocaine.

Breuer was prepared to admit that the cocaine seemed to have absolutely stopped the craving for morphine, but when Freud had begun to withdraw the cocaine, the patient started complaining. He had suffered from hallucinations and delusions, seeing snakes, dragons, and other incredible horrors.

Freud conceded lamely that he could not regard this patient's experiences as typical. But he added with a degree of firmness that he wanted the opportunity to prove that this was an unusual case. In fact, he and Dr. Koller were there to ask permission to use the hospital's laboratories and other facilities to perform tests with cocaine on human beings.

Dr. Breuer asked if they would personally conduct the tests. Freud replied that the work would be undertaken by himself and Dr. Koller with the help of a friend of the latter, Dr. Leonard Koenigstein.

KOLLER DISCOVERS
LOCAL ANESTHESIA

Carl Koller's ambition was to become an eye doctor. As the weeks of experimentation with cocaine went by, he grudgingly admitted to himself that he would rather be spending the time listening to the eye specialists—the ophthalmologists. He slipped away to attend a lecture whenever an opportunity presented.

On one such occasion, the professor had this to say: "Gentlemen, ophthalmology today has the greatest need for a new drug—for a local anesthetic. We cannot perform operations on the eye with general anesthetics, with ether, or chloroform or nitrous oxide. They are too dangerous for eye surgery; they are followed too often by nausea and vomiting, which destroy the delicate repairs on the eye. And unfortunately, too, we cannot use morphine or chloral or bromides. Until we find a compound that produces local anesthesia when dropped in the eye, we are helpless to treat cataract, iritis, and a vast number of eye diseases. . . ."[8]

This set Koller thinking. He knew that Koenigstein had attempted to cure eye infections with cocaine and had failed. He was probably right, Koller thought, in insisting that cocaine would never prevent or cure blindness. But if it could make it possible to restore sight through operations on the eye. . . .

Koller was preparing a fresh solution of cocaine as these thoughts passed through his mind. He idly flicked a few drops of the solution on his tongue.

He came back to reality with a start. His tongue had gone

numb. He touched its tip with his teeth. No feeling. He pinched his tongue with his fingers. No feeling. He called out to Koenigstein, who was in the next room, that he had discovered a local anesthetic for the eye.

Koenigstein retorted that he was crazy, but he listened nonetheless when Koller reminded him that they had always known that cocaine produced local insensitivity. The fact was generally known, but no one did anything about it.

Koenigstein asked if he had tried cocaine on the eye. The reply was that he hadn't but that he was going to right away.

They quickly got hold of some frogs and guinea pigs. Koller carefully squirted a drop of cocaine solution into one eye of a green frog squirming in the grip of a lab assistant. He instructed the young man to hold the frog carefully so that none of the solution might run into its other eye.

About two minutes were allowed to elapse. Then Koller picked up a probe and moved it toward the frog's *untreated* eye. At the first touch the frog tried desperately to move away. Koller turned to the eye in which the cocaine solution had been dropped. He touched its surface with his probe. No reaction. He pushed harder. Nothing happened. Finally, he scratched the eye firmly. The frog made no effort to escape.

He had an equal success with guinea pigs. His notebook tells the story:

"For first minute, slight irritation; animal blinks, contracts eyelids.

"Anesthesia starts immediately after, lasts approximately ten minutes with three drops of 2 percent cocaine solution.

"During anesthesia animal shows no sign of pain from following tests: needle scratch on eye, puncture of eye, cautery with silver nitrate, deep incision."[9]

Animal after animal was tested. There was no questioning the fact that cocaine produced a complete loss of sensation at the site of the application. It was time to test the human eye.

COCAINE
AND SURGERY

Koller elected himself human guinea pig. He stood quietly while Koenigstein dropped cocaine solution into his eye. He offered neither resistance nor reaction when Koenigstein and other doctors touched the usually sensitive cornea with the head of a pin.

At that time, when cataracts had to be removed, the operation was done without anesthesia. The doctors worked while the patients cried out in pain.

The next time a cataract was to be removed at the eye clinic, Koller arranged to anesthetize the patient's eye with cocaine. The surgeons were not told what he had done. They arrived, steeled as usual against the patient's inevitable cries of pain. To their amazement he sat smiling and perfectly comfortable while they cut the blinding film from the eye.

Koller's next step was to persuade Dr. Edmund Jellinek to spray the throats of patients with cocaine solution prior to surgery. The operations proved painless. Freud, who had been on vacation in Holland during these events, returned to find that Carl Koller had become famous overnight.

The German Ophthalmological Society was about to meet in Heidelberg. It was suggested that Koller attend and present his findings. But the young intern had no money for railroad fares, hotel rooms, and meals. However, his good friend Joseph Brettauer (1835-1905) of Trieste was planning to attend the meeting. Koller asked him to take his place.

The opening of the regular meeting was set for September 16, 1884. The preceding day, Dr. Brettauer called together a distinguished company. It included Professor Ferdinand Ritter von Arlt of Vienna, Professor Otto Becker of the Heidelberg staff, Dr. Henry D. Noyes of New York, and Dr. Henry Ferrer from San Francisco.

"Gentlemen," Dr. Brettauer began, "I have been asked to present you a paper which was prepared by a friend of mine in Vienna. He is Dr. Carl Koller, who is intern and house surgeon at the General Hospital. His experiments are so startling we thought it would be better to describe them first to a small group. Now if you will permit me, I shall first read Dr. Koller's manuscript. He says:

" 'It is a well-known fact that the alkaloid cocaine . . . makes the mucous membrane of the throat and mouth insensitive. . . . This led me to investigate the action of the agent on the eye. I have reached the following conclusions. . . .' "[10]

A description of the experiments on frogs and guinea pigs, the first application of cocaine solution to the human eye, and the first eye operation with cocaine followed.

Dr. Brettauer finished reading and, as he laid aside the manuscript, he suggested to the assembled leaders of the profession that their reactions were probably very much like his had been when he first read the report. It sounded impossible, and he had therefore arranged to show them exactly what cocaine could do.

A patient came in and Dr. Brettauer applied cocaine solution to one eye, nothing to the other. He then probed and pressed the treated eye. He rubbed the surface of the cornea. He spread apart the eyelids as widely as possible. He grabbed the eyeball with a forceps and pulled it back and forth.

He asked the patient if what he had been doing had hurt. The patient answered that he had felt nothing.

But when Dr. Brettauer delicately touched the eye that had not been treated, the patient flinched in pain.

His distinguished audience watched in silence. Then they loudly applauded what they had seen.

A month later Carl Koller had the gratification of personally presenting his report to the Vienna Medical Society.

There was, of course, more to the boon that Carl Koller had bestowed on mankind than its dramatic effect on eye surgery. There were the everyday occurrences in the industrial centers of large towns. Early in this century it was common for a stream of workmen to present themselves at the local dispensary with foreign bodies in their eyes. The physician on duty would insert a few drops of cocaine hydrochloride between the lids. Moments later the offending body was painlessly removed and the men returned to work as if nothing had happened.

Freud and Koller had set out to substantiate Freud's claim that cocaine was nonaddictive. This was a lost cause. But if the investigation had not been undertaken, the development of local anesthesia might have been delayed.

COCAINE
SPREADS TO AMERICA

Carl Koller moved to America and settled in New York City in 1888. His fame and the local anesthetic he had developed preceded him. American doctors were already discovering the remarkable things that could be done with cocaine.

A Norwalk, Connecticut, farmer shot himself through the hand while cleaning his revolver. He waited a day (for the bullet to fall out) before going to Dr. W. C. Burke, Jr. By that time the hand was swollen and painful.

Dr. Burke had recently read about cocaine as a local anesthetic. He injected cocaine solution into the nerve trunk from which the nerves spread throughout the hand. Five minutes later he made the long, deep incision necessary to removing the bullet. The farmer felt no pain. Thus Dr. Burke was the first to use a nerve-block procedure.

But he was only first by a matter of days. Drs. Richard John Hall (d. 1900) and William Stewart Halsted (1852-1922) of New York were right behind him when they injected cocaine into a nerve high up in a patient's leg in order to produce numbness in the entire foot.

Dr. Hall has another claim to fame. He was responsible for the introduction of local anesthesia into dentistry. His own teeth being extremely sensitive, he persuaded his dentist to use cocaine while drilling them.

Halsted for his part might have gone on to make the improvements credited to a student of his named James Leonard Corning (1855-1923). When a book by Corning on cocaine anesthesia appeared, Halsted wrote to William Osler that it was based entirely on his, Halsted's, work. ". . . I published 3 or 4 little papers in 1884-5 . . . on cocaine anesthesia," he said. "They are not creditable papers, for I was not in good form at the time."[11] Halsted was not in good form at the time because he had become addicted to cocaine while experimenting on himself. He broke the habit by having himself locked in his cabin during a long sea voyage on a private yacht. His cure seems to have been complete. In 1889 William Osler and Dr. William Henry Welch, founder of the medical school at Johns Hopkins University in Baltimore, confirmed him for the chair of surgery at that school.

Whether Halsted's claims were valid or a pipe dream, James Leonard Corning is recognized as the greatest contributor to the advancement of cocaine in the field of local anesthesia. His investigations led in two major directions.

He recognized the medical potential of the nerve-block procedure discovered by Burke, Hall, and Halsted. But he also recognized its immediate limitations. Chief of these, which he discovered by injecting his own arm with cocaine, was that the anesthesia was only effective for about twenty minutes. This obviously ruled out the use of cocaine anesthesia for any lengthy surgical procedure. Corning wondered if there was any means by which effectiveness might be prolonged. Among other experiments, he tried wrapping a tight band about his arm and injecting cocaine below the bandage. He found that anesthesia now persisted for nearly five hours. Immediate practical application of his discovery was limited. But it led later to the important discoveries of Dr. Heinrich Braun (1862-1934) of Leipzig.

Corning's second line of investigation involved the local anesthetization of the spinal cord. He injected a few drops of cocaine solution in the crevice between a dog's vertebrae. Within minutes, the entire rear end of the animal—hind legs, buttocks, tail, and thighs—was completely insensitive. His work in this area was picked up in 1899 by Rudolph Matas, the first American to report on true spinal anesthesia. The 1904 discovery of novocaine by the German chemist Alfred Einhorn (1857-1917) added safety and increased popularity to spinal anesthesia.

Meanwhile, the injection of cocaine into tissue to achieve local anesthesia had been demonstrated by Carl Schleich before the German Congress of Surgeons in 1892. Five years later, George Washington Crile, who would subsequently found the Cleveland (Ohio) Clinic, painlessly amputated a leg after injecting the sciatic and crural nerves with cocaine.

These men, from Koller in 1884 to Einhorn in 1904, were responsible for the increasing use of cocaine as an anesthetic. But they may not have been the first to use it. There is evidence to suggest that the Incas used coca-leaf infusions or extracts, introduced rectally into the body, while perforating the skull to reduce pressure on the brain. Many tombs in the Ollaechea valley of Peru have been found to contain enema syringes and a great number of trephined skulls.

COCAINE
ADDICTION

Cocaine anesthesia was being hailed as the most humane discovery in medical history to date. Cocaine was being extensively used as a supposed cure for nervous exhaustion, tuberculosis, syphilis, seasickness, and anemia, among other ills. Mariani's coca wine was in continuing demand. Mariani himself had been honored by the Pope as a benefactor of mankind. Cocaine was credited with having prolonged the life of President Ulysses S. Grant by at least four months.

Then, suddenly, American newspapers splashed headlines about "cocaine addiction."

Conservative medical men asked how this could be. Everyone *knew* that cocaine *cured* addiction. Freud rose hotly in its defense. "I can assure you that cocaine is absolutely harmless, even in long use," he wrote. "It is an absolute antidote for morphine addiction. Why, with cocaine in our hands, we can dispense entirely with asylums for addicts!"[12]

However, Freud was not as certain three years later. Having sat up many nights with his beloved friend Ernst Fleischel, a pathetic victim of cocaine, Freud withdrew his endorsement of the drug as a cure for morphine addiction. Morphine addicts are "so weak in will power, so susceptible," he wrote, that they take over cocaine as a new stimulant and replace morphine with a more destructive habit. But, he insisted, *"cocaine has claimed no other, no victim of its own."*[13] In other words, he was suggesting that no one would become a cocaine addict unless he had been a morphine addict. This was Freud's last published comment on cocaine.

There is an interesting parallel to this changing professional attitude toward cocaine in the literature of the time. Those of us who have read the Sherlock Holmes books or seen the movies will remember Holmes's frequent "Quick, Watson, the needle." Dr. Watson started giving Holmes cocaine injections after a hard day's sleuthing as early as 1886 ("A Scandal in Bohemia"). By September 1888, Holmes had become an addict. In *The Sign of the Four,* Watson says of the injections, now self-administered, "Three times a day for many months I have witnessed this performance." Holmes's addiction had reached a crisis when, in May 1891, he disappeared at Reichenbach Falls ("The Final Problem"). But Holmes no longer had a craving for cocaine when he reappeared three years later, and by 1896 we find him speaking of the hypodermic syringe as an "instrument of evil" ("The Adventure of the Missing Three-Quarter").[14]

Sir Arthur Conan Doyle, the author of the Sherlock Holmes stories, was a physician as well as a writer. It seems clear that when Conan Doyle started Holmes on the use of cocaine as a stimulant he held the professional opinion that it was harmless. The publicity about addiction forced him to turn Holmes into an addict. But the three years of "disappearance" were long enough to effect a complete cure.

General William Alexander Hammond (1828-1900) was a leader of the American medical profession, an international authority on neurology, a prolific author, and a dominant personality. He was also a strong defender of cocaine.

"There have recently been some very striking stories in the newspapers regarding the injurious effects of cocaine upon persons who have become addicted to its use," he told the Neurological Society of New York City. "In order to determine whether there was any truth in these statements, I have made some experiments on myself.

"On four different days, I gave myself an injection. And, gentlemen, I experienced none of the horrible effects, no disposition to acts of violence whatsoever; why, I didn't even want to commit a murder!

"Furthermore," Dr. Hammond continued when the laughter subsided, "I acquired no habit. I could quit its use at once. Frankly, I consider the cocaine habit, if there is such a thing, to be like the tea or coffee habit. I do not believe that there is a single instance of a well-pronounced cocaine addiction with the patient's being unable to stop at any moment he chooses to do so."

Dr. J. B. Mattison of Brooklyn was on his feet before the applause could begin. "In the past few months I have had five cocaine addicts coming to me for treatment," he announced.

Leonard Corning, the father of spinal anesthesia, quickly intervened. "There is a morbid fear of cocaine spreading through the country. Dr. Hammond's remarks have been timely and beneficial, since they seem to stop prejudice against a most useful remedy," he said.[15]

However, Dr. Mattison refused to consider himself defeated. He was joined in his seemingly hopeless battle by Alexander Shaw of St. Louis, Orpheus Everts of Cincinnati, Daniel Brower of Chicago, and Dr. Albrecht in Germany. But they were faced by ridicule and indifference. The medical profession seemed determined not to break the cocaine habit.

Help finally came from an unexpected quarter. At another New York medical meeting Dr. Frank Ring reminded those in attendance of what Dr. Hammond had had to say the previous year about giving himself four injections of cocaine without becoming addicted.

Dr. Ring announced that he had found out why Dr. Hammond did not get the habit. Four injections simply were not enough. He should have continued taking cocaine day after day for months. He should have kept on until he looked forward to it every day, until he could not wait until he had had his dose. At that point he would have had the habit all right and would not have risen at a medical meeting to tell his fellow members about it. He would have had more sense.

And then Dr. Ring concluded by saying that he was here to tell them that he was himself a cocaine addict who was unable to break the habit.

SYNTHETICS
REPLACE COCAINE

The argument for and against the possibility of cocaine addiction has been an endless one and one that may never be fully settled. To a degree, discussion has become theoretical. Half a century ago, it was common for individuals in search of mental stimulation to sniff cocaine in powder form. It was known as "nose candy." But cocaine as a means of "getting high" has been abandoned in favor of other addictive drugs, largely because it has become almost impossible to obtain (although a recent newspaper story reported the capture of an individual who was attempting to smuggle into the United States many pounds of cocaine worth tens of thousands of dollars).

Cocaine is known to inspire criminal actions. On the other hand, it can be withheld without bringing on the violent withdrawal symptoms associated with morphine and heroin. In addition, it has never been proved that coca-leaf chewing is harmful. One school of thought claims that fifty years of chewing produces no problems for the Peruvian Indians except senility. This, its adherents claim, could equally well be a product of the primitive conditions under which the natives live. But even if one accepts the proposition that there are no identifiable physical effects of chewing, there is a psychological and moral effect. The Indian survives because chewing permits him to withdraw from reality into a state of detachment, without ambition or hope for the future. Can this be called living?

After Dr. Ring made his shocking confession, physicians finally admitted that there *were* dangers in cocaine. The fact that Dr. Ring was able subsequently to break himself of the habit did not alter the picture. Scientists went in search of chemicals that would serve equally well in producing local anesthesia. They reasoned that there must be one or more that would prove safer than cocaine.

They made a fresh investigation of the coca leaf (and other plants and shrubs). It produced nothing of promise. The chemists then turned to phenol.

It was known that phenol (carbolic acid) deadened pain. Unfortunately, it also destroyed tissue. Could its formula be modified to stop tissue destruction while retaining its pain-deadening properties?

The first synthetic local anesthetic, produced by the German chemist Richard Willstätter (1872-1942) in 1902, was only the forerunner of a dozen phenol-related anesthetics. They included *orthoform, nirvanin, anesthesin, stovaine,* and *alpin.*

Then in 1904 Einhorn produced *novocaine* (procaine hydrochloride). When the United States entered World War I in 1917 and took over German patents, including that for novocaine, it was renamed *procaine.*

As the years went by, procaine replaced cocaine as a local anesthetic, except where the surface of the eye was involved. But even in eye surgery, cocaine is rarely used today. It has been replaced by such synthetics as *butyn, tetracaine,* and *lidocaine* (often found in the family medicine cabinet under the name of *xylocaine*).

ADRENALIN
AUGMENTS COCAINE

Meantime a new development opened fresh fields for the local anesthetic.

Dr. Heinrich Braun of Leipzig recalled Leonard Corning's report to the effect that, when he wrapped a tight bandage just above the site of an injection, anesthesia lasted for nearly five hours.

Dr. Braun recognized the possibility and the advantages of prolonged anesthesia, but he was forced to face the fact that one could hardly wrap a tight bandage about a man's throat when one was preparing to extract a tooth. He concluded that there must be another way.

It was clear that the bandage had operated so tightly to squeeze the blood vessels that the cocaine could not escape from the area of injection. It stayed there and continued to paralyze the sensory nerves.

What might do the same thing?

Braun considered a hundred possibilities. All of them were either ridiculous or impractical. Then he thought of *adrenalin*. Adrenalin caused blood vessels to clamp down on themselves. It constricted them as effectively as Dr. Corning's bandage.

The neck of one of Dr. Braun's patients was covered with boils. Anesthesia must be maintained for an hour if he was to open all of them without the patient feeling pain. Dr. Braun decided that here was his chance to test his theory about adrenalin.

He injected a clear solution of cocaine mixed with adrenalin into the neck and went to work on the boils. He lanced them steadily—sixteen in all. No pain! He glanced at the clock on the wall. He had been at work for an hour and ten minutes and the patient was still completely comfortable. Cocaine alone could never have done this.

COCA-COLA

The story of the coca leaf would be incomplete if something were not said about the boon it has conferred on Americans, young and old: Coca-Cola. In addition to coca, the kola nut, which contains caffeine, is used in making this beverage, hence its name.

Coca-Cola was originally developed in 1885 by John S. Pemberton of Atlanta, Georgia. He advertised it as "the intellectual beverage . . . valuable brain tonic and a cure for all nervous affections."[16]

The United States now imports hundreds of tons of coca leaf annually to be used in the manufacture of this popular drink. (Of course, the narcotic effects of cocaine are removed prior to processing!)

Wild coca, an inconspicuous greenish-brown shrub, grows abundantly in such western South American countries as Bolivia, Colombia, Ecuador, and Peru. It is also found in Australia, India, and Africa.

Coca is also grown commercially in South America, but the output has been insufficient to slake American thirst. Consequently, we encourage its cultivation in Malaya where it had never grown before. Today, the Malayan peninsula is the world's largest producer of coca leaves.

Coca is not the only plant remedy to come out of South America. The other was not a painkiller, but a cure for a scourge that has plagued mankind for several thousands of years—malarial fever.

Three

The Powder
of the Countess
⌐ Quinine

THE FEVER CAUSED
BY BAD AIR

"In the district of the city of Loxa [Loja, in Peru] grows a certain kind of large tree, which has bark like cinnamon, a little more coarse, and very bitter; which, ground to powder, is given to those who have fever, and with only this remedy, it leaves them . . ."[1]

Thus Father Calancha, an Augustinian monk living in Peru, announced to the world of 1633 a much-needed cure for malarial fever.

The existing need for a cure cannot be overestimated. A traveler journeying south from Naples in Italy and following the coastline of the Gulf of Salerno must come at length to a deserted temple standing alone in swampy wastelands. This Temple of Neptune has been rated one of the finest surviving examples of the golden age of Greek art. It was built by a colony of Greeks at Paestum, not far from modern Agropoli, Italy, around 600 B.C. The colony did well for about three hundred years. Then faulty irrigation allowed water to seep in, turning the entire area into marshlands. The Greek settlers were hard hit by fever. They blamed it on bad air (*mala aria*) rising from the marshes. They fled to higher land, leaving the Temple of Neptune as the only evidence of their having been there.

No disease, with the possible exception of bubonic plague, has more greatly changed the population distribution of the world than malaria has. This scourge has killed millions of people in Europe, Asia, Africa, and the Americas. At one time it ravaged seventeen of our southern states. Malaria has made vast areas of the world almost uninhabitable. It attacked kings, statesmen, and commoners alike—and the poor, particularly the poor.

It was characteristic of malaria that, once it took hold, it kept coming back until it ultimately killed its victim. Alexander the Great, King of Macedonia, "King of Asia," was possibly the first notable to die of malaria.

Alexander conquered Greece in the year 334 B.C. at the age of twenty-one. He was undoubtedly aided by malaria. Thanks to an abundance of water, Greece boasted some very rich and productive farmlands. But the standing water that made farming successful put forth "bad air." Everyone was attacked by fever. Those who could pull up stakes—largely the rich and the intellectuals—sought healthier places to live. The poor, the weak, the unenterprising, and the small farmers stayed where they were. Many of them died. This state of affairs had existed for many years when Alexander attacked in 334 B.C. There were few with the health and strength to resist him.

A year later, Alexander and his men were in pursuit of the army of Darius, King of the Persians. One day Alexander took a swim in a river that paralleled their line of march. He emerged with a violent chill—shivering, a cold sweat pouring from his forehead. To be smitten so rapidly, Alexander must already have been carrying the seed of malaria in his bloodstream. It would be ironic if he had picked it up in Greece.

Alexander survived this attack. In fact, over the next ten years he went on to conquer Egypt and Persia. Then, marching on India in June, 323 B.C., he was again hit by malaria. He died eleven days later.

Alexander was not the only conqueror to die of malaria. In the fifth century A.D. the barbarian king Alaric the Visigoth made the mistake of entering Rome at midsummer. The "bad air" that rose from the marshes of the Roman Campagna during the hot months was a notorious cause of fever. Alaric paid with his life.

It is interesting to note that the Pontine Marshes continued to make Rome almost uninhabitable in the summer until Mussolini drained them. His fourteen-year project was designed to reduce malaria and provide land and homes for 60,000 peasants. This was only one of several constructive projects undertaken by the misguided dictator.

Rome was not the only capital city to be plagued by malaria. It was originally intended that the residential section of Washington, D.C., would be located hard by the Capitol. This plan had to be abandoned because the swampy Anacosta River proved a hotbed of malaria. However, some fine houses had already been built when it was decided to move the residential section to higher ground in the northwest area of the city. A few of these houses still stand in the neighborhood of the Capitol.

The German leaders who succeeded Alaric tried to hold out against Rome's forbidding climate, but in the eleventh century they declared the city uninhabitable and abandoned it to the princes of the Church. The Holy Sea was to pay a heavy price in fever victims for the territory gained. Popes and cardinals died in staggering numbers. In 1241 a cardinal died at the beginning of the conclave called to elect a pope. This was a bad omen. Celestine IV, who was elected, died fifteen days after his elevation. In all, seventeen popes died from fever and other causes in the course of the thirteenth century. Six cardinals died during the conclave held in 1287.

The fourteenth century began no better. Two popes had died by 1305. However, the situation improved when Clement V moved the papal court from Rome to Avignon, France, where it remained for sixty-eight years. The move cut the papal death rate in half.

In the year 1602, malaria killed 40,000 people in Italy. By then, malaria—or ague as it was called—was spreading throughout Europe. Sir Walter Raleigh was a victim. In 1618, as he mounted the scaffold to be beheaded, he is said to have prayed that he should not be hit by an overdue attack of ague, lest his shaking and shivering be mistaken for cowardice in the face of death.

The death of James I of England seven years later has been attributed to malaria. Oliver Cromwell, lord protector of England, was a victim of the disease when he died in 1658.

Other royal persons who were attacked by malaria but survived included Charles II of England, Louis XIV of France and his son, the future Louis XV, and Maria Louisa, Queen of Spain.

EARLY ATTEMPTS
TO TREAT MALARIA

Hippocrates, the father of medicine, died twenty years before Alexander the Great was born. He had attempted to explain to the world of his day what caused the fever that held Greece helpless and horrified. He pointed out that the onset of the fever was related to the season of the year, changes in temperature, the rains, and even the direction of the wind.

Hippocrates was listing the climatic conditions that are still recognized as nature's contribution to an outbreak of malaria. What he did not of course know—nor would it be known till toward the end of the nineteenth century—was that hot weather and standing water encourage the breeding of the anopheles mosquito, the malaria carrier, while the wind dictates the direction of its attack. Understandably, Hippocrates arrived at a different and not very helpful explanation.

Fever, he said, was the result of a separation within the body of the elements of hot and cold. "So long as the hot and cold in the body are mixed together," he wrote, "they cause no pain. For the hot is tempered and moderated by the cold and the cold by the hot. But when either is entirely separated from the other, then it causes pain."[2]

According to Hippocrates, the health of an individual rested on the degree to which the four humors of the body could be kept in balance. The humors were in turn dependent on the four elements—air, earth, fire, and water. Air was the most potent of the four because it was everywhere. It was the main carrier of disease because it entered the body freely. Bad air separated the hot and the cold within the body and caused fever.

It was a neat explanation, but it did nothing to reduce the attack of fever in Greece. By the second century B.C. the population had been drastically reduced by fever. The sick began to put their faith in magic and witchcraft. This faith was no more rewarding than that of those who put their faith in doctors.

With the decline of Greece, many of her physicians moved to Alexandria in Egypt. One of them, Erasistratos of Chios, who lived at the beginning of the third century B.C., was considered a great medical authority. He disputed Hippocrates's theory of the balance of the humors. Rather, he maintained, fever was caused by blood going into the arteries which should have contained nothing but air. Therefore he tightly bound the arteries in order to stop this invasion of bad blood.

It is hard to visualize this treatment. The bound patient must have looked rather like an Egyptian mummy.

In due course, many Greek physicians gathered in Rome, the new imperial capital, some coming directly, some by way of Alexandria.

Pliny the Elder tells us that, prior to this invasion, Romans got on for six hundred years without doctors. The male head of the household looked after the diseases of his family, dependents, and slaves. Cato the Elder prescribed cabbage and wine for the relief of fever. He denounced the emigrant Greek physicians as "poisoners" and would have none of them.

The new arrivals found themselves facing their old enemy—
fever. It availed them little to blame the mists and fogs rising from
the Pontine Marshes surrounding Rome. Helpless, they resorted
to a variety of generally ineffectual forms of treatment.

A certain Petron bundled up his patients in clothes and did not
allow them to drink anything as long as the fever lasted. Since
malaria strikes during hot, often humid, weather, his "cure" must
certainly have provided a counterirritant.

Asclepiades (128-56 B.C.) of Bithynia arrived in Rome in 91
B.C. He brought with him a theory that fever was caused by atoms
blocking the pores. His method of unblocking the pores involved
diet, wine, pleasant drugs, and baths. Asclepiades must be regarded as the first of the bedside-manner school of physicians.
Such doctors give their influential patients what they figure will
make them happy, if not well. Asclepiades's motto was to heal
safely, rapidly, and pleasantly.

Andromachos of Crete was physician to the Emperor Nero.
His claim to fame lay in a concoction (which he called a theriac
or cure-all) composed of sixty-one ingredients. He prescribed his
theriac as an instant cure for fever. With sixty-one ingredients
he could hardly miss.

Pedanios Dioskorides, also practiced in the first century A.D.
He is said to have recommended *fleas* for fever. This may sound
farfetched, but no more so than a remedy favored by his contemporary, Pliny the Younger. Pliny advocated the use of eyes
of crabs, wolves, and vipers. It is not clear how these were administered.

Rufus of Ephesus (second century A.D.) offered an approach
to the fever question totally different from any other. He believed
that malarial fever could be used as a remedy for other diseases,
including epilepsy, convulsions, tetanus, asthma, melancholia, and
certain skin diseases. He wrote that there was no known drug
that heated in a more penetrating manner than fever. If, therefore, a physician were skillful enough to produce a fever arti-

ficially, it would be useless to seek other remedies against disease. His concept of fever therapy was to reappear later in medical history.

Galen (A.D. 131-201), the disciple of Hippocrates who has been held by some to have outshone his master, was born in Pergamon, Asia Minor. He reached Rome in the year 164. Understandably, he subscribed to the Hippocratic theory of the four humors. His method of restoring the loss of balance responsible for bouts of fever was purging and bleeding.

None of the fever remedies advocated by the Greek physicians turned Roman truly helped their patients.

THE NATURE
OF FEVERS

By the seventh century, the practice of medicine had fallen largely into the hands of the monks. These men of God found themselves as helpless in the face of fever as their lay predecessors had been. One of their number, the Venerable Bede, an English monk and saint, described the nature of fevers by leaning heavily on the true health given by God. He said that after the "impurity and iniquity of man's flesh which brings forth death," there will be eternal life.[3] He and other monk-physicians could only recommend prayers, exorcisms, amulets, and the ministrations of holy men as remedies for fever.

Avicenna, the eleventh-century Prince of Physicians, was equally illustrious as doctor, philosopher, scientist, statesman, and poet. His genius has been compared with that of Italy's Leonardo da Vinci (1452-1519) and Germany's Goethe (1748-1832). With a magnificence characteristic of the Arabians, Avicenna used gold, silver, and precious stones to rid the blood of impurities. Incidentally, he started a fashion for pills coated with

gold and silver dyes. He was a firm believer in the Hippocratic
theory of the humors which he gave a new lease on life.

Avicenna's fame and writing spread to Europe in the twelfth
century. The result was a European revival of the Greek school
of thought involving the humors. The monk-physicians now declared that fevers were caused by too much blood or too little
bile.

Two approaches favored by the Dominican Albertus Magnus
(*d.* 1280), teacher of St. Thomas Aquinas, might have come directly from the pages of a book on witchcraft. He regarded the
first as a remedy of sympathy because it acted at a distance from
the sick man. The prescription ran as follows: "Take the urine
of the patient and mix it with some flour to make a good dough
thereof, of which seventy-seven small cakes are made: proceed
before sunrise to an anthill and throw the cakes therein. As soon
as the insects devour the cakes the fever vanishes."[4]

The second involved direct application. Albertus "borrowed it"
from a lady of high birth who had aided many feverish persons.
"This matron of a noble family cut the ear of a cat, let three
drops of blood fall in some brandy, added a little pepper thereto,
and gave it to the patient to drink."[5]

In the fifteenth century Paracelsus upset at least a part of the
medical community by announcing that disease was caused by
chemical changes in the body rather than an imbalance in the
humors. On the whole he lost out to the followers of Hippocrates
and Galen, but his influence led some to advocate various forms
of chemotherapy. Unfortunately, Paracelsus found that the chemicals he prescribed did as little for fever as the purging and bleeding of the Galenists. In keeping with his unconventional way of
life, he then turned to magic and recommended talismans, amulets, and other witches' devices.

At the beginning of the seventeenth century, treatment for
malaria involved plasters, herbs, infusions, cordials, purging, and
bleeding. The last approach was particularly unfortunate. An

attack of malaria is accompanied by the destruction of a number of blood corpuscles. Add the deliberate withdrawal of blood and the patient winds up with an acute anemia.

All these treatments for malaria were conventional medical practices of the day. The same validity cannot be accorded astrology and witches' brews which were equally popular.

In Roman times, the Dog Star Sirius was believed to control fevers. During the so-called dog days—July 15 to August 20— this star was above the horizon at the same time as the sun. July 15 to August 20 was also the period when fever was prevalent in Rome. The connection was obvious to those who wished to make it. Now, seventeenth-century astrologers developed a system by which the course of fever could be predicted.

It involved a determination of the status of the planets at the time of the patient's birth. The "diagnosis" was complicated and was long in preparation. It cost the patient a great deal. Frequently, the fever had run its course before the diagnosis was completed. This was fortunate for the astrologer-physician since the celestial bodies that brought on the ague lacked the power to cure. About the only thing the patient received for his money was a good lesson in astrology.

When all else failed, it was always possible to blame a witch.

Finding a witch to blame was not as difficult as might be supposed. The witch had to be someone near the patient. An obvious candidate was whoever might be nursing the patient. In one case, the choice fell on a young maid who was always laughing. It did not take long to "discover" that both her mother and her grandmother had been witches. Witch-hunts have been the same through the ages. The accused is offered a chance to confess. Her fate is inevitable whether she confesses or not. There can be no doubt about the end of the laughing young maid.

Then there were the witches' brews.

A certain Dr. White led an attack on useless medicines for fever. He trained his loudest guns on Dr. Goddard's Drops. These drops were prepared from human skulls. Dr. White claimed that the skulls used were "leprous, pocky, itchy, or scrofulous." It goes without saying that Dr. White had his own exclusive remedy. It involved bleeding followed by a concoction of crabs' eyes mixed with radishes.[6]

Beyond question, the seventeenth century was ready for a tested and effective remedy for malarial fever.

THE COUNT AND COUNTESS
OF CHINCHÓN

The bark of the trees described by Father Calancha in 1633 was known as *Peruvian bark*. The name *cinchona* which is used today was conferred on it a century later by Linnaeus in his *Genera Plantarum*.

Linnaeus selected this name in honor of the Count and Countess of Chinchón, particularly the Countess. Both the Chinchóns have been credited with introducing Peruvian bark into Europe. However, there is no real evidence that they had any connection with cinchona.

Don Luis Gerónimo Fernández de Cabrera de Bobadilla Cerda y Mendoza, fourth Count of Chinchón, was a Spanish nobleman of such illustrious ancestry that he was privileged to keep his hat on in the presence of the king. The king, in this case Philip IV, appointed Chinchón viceroy of his vast South American empire. The Count ruled in Lima, Peru, from 1629 to 1640, a period which, of course, covered Calancha's discovery.

The more popular account of a Chinchón connection with cinchona involved the Countess. It claimed that she had been cured of malaria by the bark, had distributed it to malaria victims in Lima, had brought it back to Spain, and had dispensed it to feverish peasants on her husband's estates.

Unfortunately for this legend, there is no evidence that the Countess ever had malaria. Furthermore, it is quite definite that she did not return to Spain. While she, the Count, and their eleven-year-old son were waiting for the fleet that would carry them home, Doña Francisca, Countess of Chinchón, died from some unidentified disease and was buried at Cartagena, Colombia, on January 14, 1641.

On the other hand, the Count was already familiar with malaria when he journeyed to the New World. He had seen it in Madrid, in Seville, and on his own swampy farmlands.

It is uncertain whether he had himself contracted malaria before leaving Spain or whether his first attack came in Peru. But it is quite definite that he suffered many bouts during his eleven years in Lima. The record shows that the Countess represented him at public functions on a number of occasions when he was ill with fever.

Therefore it would seem that if any member of the family introduced Europe to cinchona it would have to be the Count. But whenever the Count had an attack of fever his personal physician, Don Juan de Vega, always bled him, because he knew of no other treatment. This would suggest that neither the Count nor his physician was aware of (or, if aware, believed in) the local cure for malaria.

Still, it is clear that, by whatever agent, Peruvian bark reached Europe around the time of the Count of Chinchón's return to Spain. It found immediate favor in all countries where malaria attacks were frequent—Italy, Spain, Belgium, Holland, France, and England. Early shipments from Peru sold for more than their weight in gold.

JESUITS'
POWDER

Under the name of Peruvian bark, or the "Powder of the Countess" as it was already sometimes called, the new remedy was doing a thriving business. Then the Society of Jesus began dispensing it, changing its name to *Jesuits' Powder*. Business promptly fell off. Protestants declared that they would rather die of malaria than touch Jesuits' Powder. They even claimed that its introduction was part of a diabolical plot instigated by the Pope to rid the world of non-Catholics. Oliver Cromwell, offered Jesuits' Powder on his deathbed in 1658, chose to refuse the powder and die.

Doctors may have scoffed at such superstitions on the part of laymen, but they were themselves far from free of superstitious beliefs and practices. Fourteen centuries earlier the great Galen had provided a catalogue of *all good drugs*. Why was Peruvian bark not included in the list, if it was all that it was cracked up to be, the doctors asked, preferring to overlook the fact that it had not been discovered in Galen's day. Rather than fly in the face of the traditional, it was safer to stick with such tried and true remedies as viper's broth or crab's eyes or murderer's skull. These remedies might not cure the patient, but they would not directly kill him. This approach was certainly easier than deciding to try something new.

ROBERT TALBOR,
SUCCESSFUL QUACK

Robert Talbor (1642-1681) was an exception.

Destined to become official physician to Charles II of England, Talbor was born in Cambridge a year after the Countess of Chinchón died in Colombia. His grandfather was registrar of the university. Young Robert entered St. John's College but dropped out of school in 1663 at the age of twenty-one. He then became an apprentice in the Cambridge apothecary shop of a Mr. Dent.

Among the things Talbor learned about from Mr. Dent was Peruvian bark and the medical profession's reluctance to experiment with it.

In 1666, the eminent English physician Thomas Sydenham published a book called *Method for Curing the Fever.* Syndenham was a staunch follower of Hippocrates and Galen. He firmly believed in an imbalance of the humors as the cause of illness. Sydenham pointed to the effectiveness attributed to Jesuits' Powder as proof that malarial fevers were caused by corrupt humors. But, he insisted, the powder stopped the process of fermentation by which the corrupt humors were destroyed, when it lowered the patient's temperature. This could only endanger the life of the patient. However, he grudgingly admitted that, prudently administered, the powder *might* have some beneficial effect if given *after* the fever had declined—that is, after the corrupt humors had been eliminated.

About the time that Sydenham was bestowing this kiss of death on Peruvian bark, word came from the Essex coast (an extremely marshy region infested with deadly ague) that a man there—

not a physician—was curing the fever. It was none other than Robert Talbor.

In 1668 Talbor set himself up in London as a full-fledged doctor. Then he published a little book on the art of curing malaria —by his own secret remedy.

Soon he had charmed his way through polite society into royal circles. He reached his pinnacle when he cured King Charles II of malaria. He was knighted and appointed court physician. He stood in such favor with the king that His Majesty instructed the Royal College of Physicians that its members "should not give [Talbor] any molestation or disturbance in his practice . . ."[7]

Sir Robert now had no difficulty in gaining acceptance for his "secret remedy to cure fevers" which was "a safe and worthy substitute for Peruvian bark . . . [or] . . . Jesuit's Powder [which] may be a noble medicine when given properly, but . . . has dangerous effects when administered by the unskilled. On the other hand, my remedy is always safe, it is infinitely better than Peruvian bark!"[8]

There was only one distortion in this advertisement. It appears in the final sentence. The effective ingredient in the Talbor remedy *was* Peruvian bark.

Seven years passed, during which Sir Robert boasted a near monopoly of English cures. Then word came that Louis XIV's only living son, the French dauphin, was down with malaria. The court physicians had tried everything—except, of course, Peruvian bark. The heir to the throne showed no improvement. King Charles had spent many years in exile at the French court. Louis was his dear friend. Charles sent his personal physician to Paris to take care of the fever-stricken prince. Sir Robert cured him.

Malaria was common in the Bourbon family. Louis XIV himself had had a bout forty years earlier and had been cured with Peruvian bark. (If he had recalled this, he might now have saved himself a lot of money.) He was anxious to obtain Talbor's secret formula. Sir Robert did not hesitate to name his price. He demanded the title of Chevalier, 3,000 gold crowns, a substantial pension for life, and a promise by Louis that he would not make his secret public until after his death.

The humiliated French physicians were understandably eager to discredit this English charlatan, but again he proved too much for them. They asked him, "What is fever?" "I do not know," Talbor replied. Then he added: "You gentlemen may explain the nature of fever; but I can cure it, which you cannot."[9] His cures included the Prince de Condé and the Duc de la Rochefoucauld. When the Queen of Spain became ill with fever, Louis sent Sir Robert to take care of her.

Talbor was rich as well as famous when he returned to England in 1681. But he died a few months later at the age of thirty-nine. St. John's College, Cambridge, where he had studied briefly, hailed him as an illustrious English physician and made him a fellow of the college. But, as a quack who had become famous, Talbor feared that on his death he would be repudiated by the medical profession and quickly forgotten. Therefore, to assure his immortality, he had a monument erected at Holy Trinity Church, Cambridge, where he was to be buried. It described him as the "most honourable Robert Talbor, Knight and Singular Physician, unique in curing Fevers of which he had delivered Charles II King of England, Louis XIV King of France, the Most Serene Dauphin, Princes, many a Duke and a large number of lesser personages."[10] He might have spared himself the expense. Another imposing tablet in the same church hailed him more simply as *Febrium Malleus*—smasher of fevers.

PERUVIAN BARK
FINALLY ACCEPTED

In January 1682 Louis revealed Sir Robert's secret in a book that was immediately translated into English under the title of *The English Remedy: or, Talbor's Wonderful Secret, for Cureing of Agues and Feavers.* The much-touted prescription involved six drachms of rose leaves infused for four hours with six ounces of water, two ounces of lemon juice, and a good portion of Peruvian bark. The rose leaves and lemon juice were window dressing. The active ingredient was Peruvian bark.

Up to this time, resistance to Peruvian bark had been fortified by the fact that its use would have been at odds with the classical medical beliefs still followed by many physicians. These men would rather have died (and let their patients die) than use a remedy not recommended by Galen.

Now Peruvian bark became part of an escalating challenge to Galen's hitherto largely undisputed sway. French doctors somewhat sheepishly accepted the bark that some of their predecessors had used forty years earlier.

The English soon followed suit. As mentioned earlier, in 1666 Thomas Sydenham had condemned Peruvian bark with the faint praise of possibly having some beneficial effect after the fever had subsided. Now he was one of the first to use it in his practice. He wrote: "Of all the simples, Peruvian bark is the best; for a few grains morning and evening strengthen and enliven the blood."[11] (A "simple" is a medicinal plant or a vegetable drug having only one ingredient.)

By the close of the century, Johann Conrad Peyer and Michele Bernard Valentini had formally introduced the bark into Germany and Francesco Torti had done Italy a like service. In 1711, Torti published the first complete treatise on the medicinal properties of the bark. Most importantly, he established with absolute certainty that malaria was the only type of fever that could be cured by the bark. His proof exploded a long-held theory that all fevers were caused by the same agent. If this theory had been valid, he pointed out, Peruvian bark would have been effective with all fevers. Incidentally, it was Torti who bestowed on *the ague* its modern name—*mal-aria*. He was of course prompted by the age-old belief that this fever was caused by poisonous gases arising from stagnant marshlands. This was understandable. Roughly 175 years were still to pass before anyone would know that a mosquito was the culprit.

Peruvian bark, or cinchona as it would soon be called, was finally and firmly established on the list of acceptable remedies.

THE DE LA CONDAMINE EXPEDITION

One hundred years after cinchona bark was first brought to Europe, Peru remained its only source. Many felt that it was time to break this *de facto* monopoly.

This undertaking proved more difficult than might have been anticipated. Another one hundred years would elapse before cinchona was successfully grown outside of South America.

Charles de la Condamine (1701-1774), naturalist, mathematician, and explorer, was third in command of the French scientific expedition that arrived in Quito, Ecuador, in 1735 to verify the shape of the earth. History, however, identifies it as the de la Condamine expedition.

One, if not both, of de la Condamine's superiors was a more accomplished scientist. But whatever de la Condamine may have lacked professionally was made up by showmanship. He was charming, witty, sophisticated, widely read, and capable of using his pen like a rapier. He was an intimate of statesmen and at home in the salons of duchesses. However, the very qualities that would later lead to the identification of the expedition with his name were undoubtedly the cause of the disagreements that decided de la Condamine seven years later to break with his associates and head south by way of the Andes. Soon he found himself in the lush cinchona forests of Loja.

There is little reason to suppose that de la Condamine set out on his lonely journey with cinchona in mind. However, an encounter with a bark trader revealed how very little was paid for the bark at its source in contrast with the exorbitant price it fetched in Europe. He decided to take cinchona trees to France and raise them there. His motivation was certainly the prospect of substantial profits, but he was not unmindful of the fact that success would mean a crack in the monopoly.

De la Condamine collected a large number of seedlings, planted them in boxes of earth, and set off across the mountains in the direction of the Amazon River. He and his Indian companions safely carried the seedlings across swamps and jungles, avoiding hostile natives and dangerous animals, and then through the wild rapids of the untamed river. The trip took eight months.

The end was in sight. In a matter of hours de la Condamine would board the ship that would take him and his precious cargo to France. Suddenly, a huge wave swamped his craft. De la Condamine escaped with his life, but his plants were gone.

On his return to France in 1745 after spending ten years in the New World de la Condamine was physically battered, full of infirmities, and totally deaf. But his mind and his tongue remained as quick as ever.

Another member of the de la Condamine expedition was Joseph de Jussieu who classified *Erythroxylon coca*. His primary objective in joining the expedition was to get to Peru and study the cinchona tree.

De Jussieu spent seventeen years traveling far and wide in the South American jungles and up and down the Andes in search of cinchona. He taught botany, practiced medicine, designed bridges and dams, and built roads in order to support himself. Meanwhile he was studying an infinite variety of plants, animals, and minerals and the customs of the various Indian tribes. He made careful maps wherever he went. He acquired a wealth of scientific material that European scientists of his day had never dreamed of. He stored his incredible accumulation of information in locked wooden boxes that were watched over night and day by a trusted servant.

When he finally decided to return to France in 1761, like de la Condamine sixteen years earlier, he was determined to bring home the cinchona tree. However, he selected seeds rather than seedlings, packing them in yet another wooden strongbox.

As the day for de Jussieu's departure from Buenos Aires neared, the "trusted" servant decided that the boxes he had been required to watch over so carefully must be filled with precious stones. Seizing one of the rare occasions when de Jussieu let the boxes out of his sight, he made off with them. One can imagine the thief's disgust when he pried them open and found nothing but worthless seeds and papers, which he doubtless scattered to the wind. Another attempt to bring the cinchona tree to Europe had failed just as success seemed assured.

De Jussieu did not return to France. No one knows where he was or what happened to him during the next ten years. He was hopelessly insane when he finally reached Paris in 1771.

There seems to have been a jinx on the transportation and raising of cinchona trees. De la Condamine and de Jussieu were not alone in failure. A Jesuit expedition succeeded in transporting seedlings to Algeria but they died after arriving at their new home.

Seed carried to Paris and Java by French and Dutch expeditions failed to germinate.

Finally, another obstacle was added to those already faced by would-be collectors. Peruvian authorities decided to convert their long-enjoyed *de facto* monopoly into a *de jure* monopoly. They placed the cinchona forests off limits to foreigners. Those who attempted to penetrate them were subject to stiff penalties.

PELLETIER
AND CAVENTOU
DEVELOP QUININE

Powdered cinchona bark was recognized as the only known cure for malarial fever. The next step was to find out what specific substance in the bark was responsible for the cure. Obviously, reliable dosage could not be achieved until this element was isolated. Powdered bark contained impurities. Its performance was erratic, to say the least. The situation was similar to that of the first opium encountered by Sertuerner that had headed him in the direction of morphine.

Two Frenchmen, Pierre Joseph Pelletier (1788-1842), a twenty-nine-year-old professor of pharmacy, and Joseph Bien-aimé Caventou (1795-1877), a twenty-two-year-old pharmacy student, met for the first time in 1817. Both had read Sertuerner's recently published full report of his work on morphine. They were impressed by the simplicity and directness of his approach. They concluded that they should be able to extract the active ingredients of other plants, just as he had extracted morphine from opium.

They first tackled ipecac, an import from South America used to induce vomiting and as a cure for dysentery and diarrhea. Pelletier and Caventou isolated its pure chemical and called it *emetine.* Next they produced *strychnine* from the poisonous *Strychnos* plant of Sardinia.

It was clear that emetine and strychnine were members of a new family of chemicals to which Sertuerner's morphine also belonged. All were plant products that performed very much like alkalies. A German chemist, Meissner, gave them the name of *alkaloids.*

Pelletier and Caventou—and others—extracted a number of different alkaloids from a number of different plants. Apart from being alkaloids, these seemed to have only one thing in common —they had little or no commercial value.

At the time he was collaborating with Pelletier, Caventou was also studying under the eminent French chemist Louis-Jacques Thénard (1777-1857). One day Thénard instructed another student to prepare an extract of cinchona for class demonstration. The student casually commented to Caventou that the cinchona extract he had produced seemed extremely alkaline.

This was enough for Caventou. He rushed to Pelletier and suggested that they start work at once on cinchona. The older man wanted to know why cinchona rather than other possible sources. It was true that cinchona cured malaria, which was claiming thousands of victims each year, but so were tuberculosis, plague, and smallpox. What was so special about malaria and cinchona?

Caventou told what his fellow student had found and concluded that there might be an alkaloid in cinchona. This was the clincher, and he and Pelletier went to work.

Many men—in Sweden, France, Germany, Scotland, and Portugal—had attempted to isolate the active element in cinchona bark. They had found chemicals that were new to them but none that had the slightest curative effect on malaria. However, none of these researchers had been looking for an alkaloid. In fact, they had not known that alkaloids existed.

It had taken Sertuerner a year to isolate morphine. Pelletier and Caventou produced white crystals from an extract of gray cinchona in a matter of days. Unfortunately, their fine white crystals were no cure for malaria.

Pelletier was ready to drop the investigation then and there. Fortunately the irrepressible Caventou recalled a book in which a doctor had said that not all cinchona barks are the same and different barks have varying effects on malaria. They had been working with gray bark. He proposed that they try yellow bark.

They did not get the shiny white crystals they had been expecting and hoping for. All they got was a sticky, pale yellow gum that would not crystallize whatever they did. The gum was soluble in acid, alcohol, and ether and was definitely a new chemical. They called it *quinine* from an old Peruvian Indian name for the bark —*quinaquina*.

Quinine was the active element in cinchona—pure, potent, and dependable. Unfortunately, it cost so much to produce that it was only available to the very rich.

THE DUTCH GO AFTER
CINCHONA

By 1853 the Dutch were set to make another attempt to break the South American monopoly. Early that year they sent one of their most distinguished botanists, Justus Charles Hasskarl (1811-1894), to Peru. It was expected that Hasskarl would run into trouble. He did. He played hide-and-seek with officials up and down the Andes, trying to get into the forests to collect seeds at the proper time. He bribed officials and paid natives to collect seed for him. He held secret meetings near the Bolivian border. At these, bags of gold were exchanged for bags of seed.

He changed his name frequently, actually arriving in Peru with the identity and credentials of José Carlos Muller. The governor of Sina introduced "Herr Muller" to a dubious character named

Henriquez. The governor had refused a direct offer of money but Henriquez was ready to produce cinchona plants from the forest of Carabaya at a fancy price.

Hasskarl dragged these plants and his bags of seed by jungle path 150 miles to Arequipa. It was no easy journey. He then made the port of Islay where the frigate *Prins Frederik de Nederlanden* was waiting for him and his precious cargo.

Hasskarl reached Java in December 1854. The cinchona plants had died during the voyage but there were still thousands of seeds. The seeds were planted; they sprouted. In time there were cinchona trees. Success at last—or so the Dutch thought.

But the bark of these trees contained no quinine. Hasskarl was only one among many who did not know that there were some fifty kinds of cinchona trees of which only a few produce quinine. Hasskarl had acquired the seeds of the wrong kinds of trees.

The Dutch had dreamed of mass-produced quinine, but this dream had faded and with it the relief that might have been brought to the suffering poor.

Still there was worse to come.

An investigator named Antonio Ullca had warned the Indians that wholesale stripping of bark would kill the cinchona trees. The natives had paid no attention to him and now the cinchonas were close to extinction in many parts of Peru. Scarcity further drove up the price of Peruvian bark.

Fortunately, cinchona forests were discovered in neighboring Bolivia, Ecuador, and Colombia. The authorities of these countries were determined that the industry should not fall into the hands of foreigners. Under their strict regulations, dead bark might be exported but not seeds or living plants. The monopoly remained intact and, with Peruvian production virtually at a standstill, the price of cinchona bark went up and up.

THE BRITISH
MAKE THEIR BID

The government of British India had long considered the possibility of raising cinchona trees locally. After all, the demand for quinine in the subcontinent was immense.

In 1859 Clements Robert Markham (1830-1916), a twenty-nine-year-old clerk in a London governmental office, laid before the revenue committee of the India Office a plan to collect cinchona seeds and plants and introduce them into India and Ceylon.

Markham's plan was quickly approved. It was an elaborate, well-constructed plan. It involved four separate expeditions operating along a 2000-mile front in remote, isolated areas rather than a single unit. The four expeditions would move in rapidly, without fanfare, and all at the same time. Markham had no illusions about the difficulties they would face in trying to avoid being turned back or apprehended by the authorities. But he felt it was a good gamble that at least one of the units would succeed. In point of fact all of them did.

Markham chose for himself the surviving yellow-bark cinchona of southern Peru. He was accompanied by a young English gardener named Weir. They found that local determination to stem the foreign assault on cinchonas did not lessen as they climbed higher and higher into the Andes.

In a shepherd's hut many thousands of feet above sea level where they spent a night they met Don Manuel Martel, a former colonel in the Peruvian army. He seemed friendly enough, and it was understandable that the conversation would turn to cinchona. He spoke of José Muller, an evil Dutchman who had stolen cinchona plants. He accused him of robbing the peasants of their living. Never having heard of Hasskarl by this name, Markham and Weir could truthfully declare that they did not know him. Martel seemed satisfied when they assured him that their own interests did not include cinchona and that they were actually headed away from the banned forests.

The next morning they went their separate ways. However, as soon as Martel was well along the path for the city of Puno on Lake Titicaca, Markham and Weir headed upward toward the Carabaya valley with its forests of cinchona trees.

It had taken a month to reach the valley. It took another month to collect seedlings and make preparations for a start back to the coast. Then early one morning they loaded their mules with their precious seedlings wrapped in matting and started down trail.

It became apparent the first time they stopped at a settlement that Colonel Martel had had second thoughts about them and had given orders to detain them. Not only were the inhabitants no longer friendly, but they would provide the foreigners with provisions and fresh pack animals only if they agreed to return as they had come, via Puno. It was easy to guess what sort of reception committee would be awaiting them there.

They had no choice but to seem to agree. They ostentatiously started toward Puno with all the animals. What the natives did not know was that these were loaded with only a few of the cinchona plants. The rest were on the backs of three animals Markham had stolen and hidden. As soon as they were well out of sight of the settlement, Markham doubled back, retrieved the hidden mules, and lit out by a different route for Arequipa, the city two days' march from the coast that had been their jumping-off place.

His plan was to follow a straight-line course over the Andes. It was a crazy undertaking with only a compass and the crudest of maps to guide him. Nevertheless he marched safely into Arequipa ten days after he separated from Weir.

The gardener joined him there two days later. He had been

stripped of his few seedlings but had been able to talk Martel into letting him go. Perhaps the colonel though he would lead him to Markham and a richer prize. If so, he was disappointed. Markham and Weir had no difficulty in making Punta Islay and the British consulate where they had left miniature greenhouses, al-ready filled with soil, in which to carry home whatever plants they might collect.

An explorer named Pritchett led the second expedition. His assignment was to collect gray-bark cinchonas in the Huánuco forests of central Peru lying north of Lima. He was as successful as Markham. He brought out his collection of gray-barks a few months after Markham's return to Arequipa.

The objective of Dr. Richard Spruce, a distinguished botanist, was the red-bark cinchonas of the Ecuadorian Andes. This was no easy assignment. Spruce was faced with a three-month trip through the region of the head-hunting Jivaros and up the walls of Chimborazo, the highest peak in the Cordillera Real.

The trip would have been rigorous for a man in his prime. This Spruce had never been. One morning he woke with a paralytic condition in his back and legs. "From that day forth," he wrote later, "I was never able to sit up straight or to walk about without great pain and discomfort, soon passing to mortal exhaustion."[12] Nevertheless, he dragged himself across torrents and up moun-tains until he saw what he described as the most beautiful tree in the world. The red-barked cinchonas looked like a royal carpet on the slopes of Chimborazo.

A civil war was raging in Ecuador. No manual help was ob-tainable. Aided only by one of Markham's botanists, Spruce managed to collect 100,000 seeds and get them off safely to England.

But the price he personally paid was great. He was forty-three when he came out of the forests. The severe rheumatism and intermittent paralysis he had contracted there turned him into a helpless invalid. He lived another thirty-three years of which the final twenty were spent flat on his back. All his life he had had nothing but what he earned. In his forced retirement he was left penniless.

The fourth Markham expedition was led by a Scotsman named Cross. He brought crown bark out of Ecuador and Colombian barks out of Colombia.

Markham's gamble had paid off beyond all expectations. The seeds and seedlings that were gathered reached India in 1860 and were planted there and in Ceylon. Six years later the plantations were providing the London market with a good supply of quinine. Then insects attacked and destroyed all but the red cinchonas. These provided too small a yield of quinine to make them competitive with other South American barks. The Indian and Singhalese planters abandoned cinchona in favor of tea.

THE DUTCH PRODUCE
QUININE IN JAVA

Charles Ledger, an Englishman, had lived in Peru for many years. He knew cinchona better than most botanists. Hearing of Markham's expeditions, Ledger decided to collect and sell him calisaya bark. This particular bark offered the greatest quinine yield of all. His servant Manuel had been with him for sixteen years. He asked Manuel where the "true bark" grew. Only, his servant told him, "where the trees could see the snow-capped mountains."

The white man had sought the calisaya for two hundred years. Manuel's people had kept them way from it. Now Manuel agreed to gather seed for his master.

He went into the mountains. He did not come out again for five years. He had been waiting for the "best crop," he explained. However, he had now brought his master fourteen pounds of seed worth a small fortune.

It was 1865. Markham had been and gone. Ledger sent his seed to England for sale to the British government. It was not interested. The Indian venture had not yet failed, and there was more than enough seed from Markham's expeditions.

The Dutch were equally indifferent at first. In the end, they bought one pound for 100 gulden with the understanding that Ledger would be further compensated if the seed proved fertile.

When the small box containing the seed was opened in Java, the smell of decay was so strong that it seemed certain that the seeds were rotten. But they germinated readily and Ledger received 500 gulden more. His one pound of seed was the basis for the thriving Dutch cinchona industry in Java.

The Indian and Singhalese ventures had been abandoned by the time the Java bark became marketable. The Dutch established a monopoly of their own, but of a different type. The South Americans had used their monopoly to drive the price of quinine up; the Dutch used their abundant crops to hold it down.

The approach was commercially sound. The low price discouraged competition. There was no incentive for the likes of Markham to face hardships of forest collecting. At the same time, quinine was brought within the reach of the many malaria sufferers rather than the few. The monopoly was based on quantity.

WARBURG'S
TINCTURE

Their dream of locally produced quinine having faded, the British in India turned to publicized remedies. A favorite was Warburg's Tincture, a "secret" cure produced by an Austrian physician. One British general stationed at Mysore bought 1,500 bottles at his own expense for distribution to his troops.

In 1875, the Inspector General of the British Army reported

in the British medical journal *The Lancet* that he had been called upon to treat fever of all degrees in India, China, and the Gold Coast and that nothing had proved as effective as Warburg's Tincture. He then revealed the formula: aloes, rhubarb, camphor, and various herbs mixed with *a liberal amount of sulphate of quinine.*

MALARIA
IN AMERICA

Most people associate malaria with dark, remote parts of the world. However, malaria was a common and serious threat to the inhabitants of the Mississippi Valley and a strong deterrent to westward migration as recently as 150 years ago. Political enemies claimed that Thomas Jefferson's Louisiana Purchase of 1803 had bought only a vast amount of uninhabitable land.

It seems unlikely that the American Indian suffered from malaria. This would suggest that the disease came from Africa with the slaves. In this connection it must be realized that some malarial parasites can remain in a victim's bloodstream for as long as thirty years. So long·as the Indians were malaria-free, the anopheles mosquitoes of the Mississippi Valley remained malaria-free. But when malaria-infested slaves were bitten by these mosquitoes, long dormant parasites turned the mosquitoes into malaria carriers. (This process was repeated in recent years when Vietnam veterans brought home to the southern states malarial strains new to the local mosquito population.)

It was John Sappington (1776-1856), a country doctor, who transformed Jefferson's "wilderness" into a home for forty million people. His solution was to clean out the malaria. His achievement becomes all the more remarkable when we remember that the malarial parasite was not uncovered by Charles Laveran, the

French physiologist and bacteriologist, until 1880, twenty-four years after Sappington's death. Furthermore, the English pathologist Sir Ronald Ross (1857-1932) did not identify the mosquito as the carrier until 1897. Like men of science and medicine centuries before him, Sappington attributed the ague known as malaria to some noxious agent in the air.

Sappington was born in Maryland but later the family moved to Nashville, Tennessee. Here John served a five-year apprenticeship with his physician-father and then joined him in practice.

By 1819 John Sappington had established himself and his family in a log-cabin home called Arrow Rock near where the Santa Fe Trail left the Missouri River in Saline County, Missouri. It was shortly thereafter that the frightening potential of malaria was recognized.

In 1820 an Ohio newspaper waxed poetic in reporting that "the angel of disease and death, ascending from his oozy bed, along the marshy margins of the bottom grounds . . . floats in his aerial chariot, and in seasons favorable to his progress, spreads mortal desolation as he flies."[13] Two years later, an Indianapolis physician revealed that 90 percent of his patients had been smitten by fever at the same time.

Whole villages in Michigan were paralyzed. The few villagers who survived the malarial epidemic were said to "crawl about like yellow ghosts." The situation became so bad that a popular jingle offered this warning:

> Don't go to Michigan, that land of ills;
> The word means ague, fever and chills.[14]

Malaria was so universal in the Great Plains that it became customary to say: "He ain't sick, he's only got the ague." Daniel Drake (1785-1852), a famous Midwestern medical contemporary of Sappington, rated malaria the most important disease in the Mississippi Valley.

Cinchona bark had been used as a fever-fighter for several centuries but it was mostly given in small doses *after* the fever was reduced. A year after Sappington settled at Arrow Rock, Pelletier and Caventou, as mentioned earlier, isolated the alkaloid quinine. The first American quinine factory was established in Philadelphia two years later.

Before this, malaria was attacked by Benjamin Rush and other Philadelphia physicians with purgings, induced vomiting, and blood-letting. The effect of such treatment was to further weaken patients already debilitated by fever. The quinine treatment was certainly more humane and more effective. But with quinine now readily available, even as progressive a doctor as Daniel Drake hesitated to give up purgatives and the knife. Henry Perrin is said to have harbored like reservations, but he is nonetheless credited with being the first to use large doses of quinine at the first signs of malarial fever.

Sappington, for his part, adopted quinine as his *sole* method of treating malaria soon after it became commercially available in 1823. Nine years later he was manufacturing and distributing the quinine pills that were to make him famous.

Sappington got into the pill business by accident. He had sent one of his sons to Philadelphia to buy 100 ounces of quinine. The young man returned with 100 pounds, almost all the quinine then available in the country.

To recoup what was to this country doctor a shattering investment, Sappington decided to make and sell pills. His formula called for quinine sulphate, licorice, and myrrh (in the proportion of 4 to 3 to 1), with oil of sassafras as a flavor additive. Initial sales were spectacular. Sappington taught his slaves how to manufacture the pills. A box containing twenty-four pills cost about ten cents to manufacture and sold for $1.50. It is estimated that Sappington sold more than a million pills.

Sales were not entirely dependent on the testimonials that poured in from grateful purchasers. Sappington must be recognized as the father of audio-advertising. In earlier days a bell on the roof of Arrow Rock Tavern had warned of Indian raids. Now Dr. John began to give it a clang every evening to remind folks to take their pills. This practice spread from community to community over the Great Plains as salesmen journeyed through them with pills, books, and handbills. Incidentally, Sappington required his salesmen to take one quinine pill three times a day. It is reported that not even those who traveled through areas where malaria was most prevalent ever contracted the disease.

Sappington's program was built on a false premise. Certain chemicals will prevent certain forms of malaria, but quinine is not one of them. Quinine does, however, operate to suppress the symptoms by which malaria is recognized. The supposed immunity of Sappington's salesmen and other regular pill-takers was more a matter of good faith and fortune than of good preventive medicine.

How unfortunate an attempt to use quinine as a preventive can prove was revealed by a report made in 1900. After noting that as much as 200,000 ounces was used annually to control malarial fever during early work on the Panama Canal, H. A. Martin, the writer of the report, continues: "Many of the employees were in the habit of taking as a prophylactic [preventive measure] *large* doses of the drug in rum or vermouth every morning before breakfast—a teaspoonful, in fact, was looked upon as a small dose. The consequence was that when the attack did come the only medicine that might have proved effective to save life was powerless, as the system had become so tolerant of its action."[15]

SYNTHETIC DRUGS
REPLACE QUININE

Quinine cured malaria, but no one knew why; in fact, no one really knew what caused malaria. Then in 1879 things began to happen.

Patrick Manson (1844-1922), the British "father of tropical medicine," discovered that filariasis, an infection much like malaria, was spread by mosquitoes. Four years later, Alfred Freeman Africanus King wrote an article for *Popular Science Monthly* in which he gave nineteen reasons for believing that malaria was transmitted by the bite of a mosquito. It took Ronald Ross, whose work would be rewarded with a Nobel prize in 1902, eleven more years to identify the strange microbe that spent part of its life in the anopheles mosquito and part in human blood. He went on to demonstrate that quinine destroys the malaria germ in human blood.

Engineers, public health officials, and sanitary experts went to work to wipe out the mosquito, but their success was necessarily limited. There was still a demand for quinine, and it soon became obvious that filling this demand called for a synthetic substitute for quinine.

German scientists were already at work on the structure of the quinine molecule. As early as 1879 Z. H. Skraup had identified *quinoline*. A few years later Wilhelm Koenigs uncovered *meroquine*. In 1907, P. Rabe and Heinrich Hoerlein established the fact that the complete quinine molecule involved a quinoline unit and a meroquine unit tied together by a simple alcohol unit. Obviously the malaria-killing power of quinine must lie in one of these units. They were tried singly and in combination, but nothing worked to kill the malaria germ.

Still, there had to be an answer.

Schulemann of the great German Dye Trust kept after quinoline. He took it apart and put it back together again. He found that by attaching a long tail of carbon atoms he could turn a mild chemical into a substance that completely destroyed malaria germs. He called this substance *plasmoquine*. Unfortunately, it soon became apparent that plasmoquine, while killing malaria germs, could also kill their human hosts.

Back to the test tubes. It took roughly another ten years to produce *atabrine* (later to be called *quinacrine*). Here at last was a chemically produced cure for malaria that not only worked but produced minimal side effects. The worst that could be said of it was that it occasionally caused a temporary yellow discoloration of the skin and sometimes indigestion and stomach distress. Meanwhile British and American scientists had joined the search.

Two synthetic drugs produced in 1939 were considered by many public health physicians to be superior to quinine. One, developed at the Liverpool School of Tropical Medicine, was marketed throughout England and the Far East under the name of *chloroguanide hydrochloride*. The second was discovered at Johns Hopkins University Laboratory for Tropical Disease, Baltimore. It was sold under the name of *chloroquine phosphate*.

At the outbreak of World War II several U.S. pharmaceutical houses began to manufacture German synthetic drugs. Among them was quinacrine hydrochloride (atabrine). The United States also made available for commercial use a German formula of chlorophenothane (DDT) that effectively destroyed 85 to 90 percent of the mosquito population.

Japan came into possession of the chief source of quinine when she took over the Dutch colonies in Southeast Asia during World War II. Fortunately, the United States had bought 13 million ounces of quinine from the Dutch several years earlier. This supply and the expanding production of effective synthetic drugs were used to treat the combat troops of America and her allies in the malaria-infested areas of Asia and the South Pacific.

The synthetic drugs in use then are generally the ones in use today.

But quinine, in pure or synthetic form, was a cure for malarial fever only. What about other fevers?

The standard family remedy for everyday fever has its own fascinating story.

Four

*The Remedy
in Every Medicine Cabinet*
⌐ Aspirin

WILLOW BARK
AS A FOLK REMEDY

Aspirin is a household word. There is scarcely a person in the United States, child, teenager, or adult, who has not heard of it. Television sings its praise as a painkiller—aspirin alone or in combination with other drugs. There is scarcely a person, child, teenager, or adult, who has not taken aspirin. It is in every family medicine cabinet. There is even special aspirin for young children.

Aspirin—or acetylsalicylic acid, to give its full chemical name —is a white crystalline solid formed by the action of acetic anhydride on salicylic acid. Today, salicylic acid is obtained from phenol—a coal-tar derivative. But this has not always been the case. The original source of salicylic acid was the bark of the willow tree. The botanical name for willows is *Salix,* from which we have arrived at *salicylic.*

Salicylic acid obtained from phenol is no better than that obtained from willow bark. We use the synthetic product rather than that occurring in nature because it is cheaper to produce.

The use of salicylic acid in the treatment of pain and fever is far from new. There are records that show that the Romans were obtaining it from willow-tree bark and using it as early as 400 B.C. Also, our pioneers pushing westward found that the North American Indians had long used a willow bark as a remedy.

But, as is usually the case, these early users of what would someday be aspirin knew what the natural product did but not why it did it. That knowledge did not come until the nineteenth century.

THE SEARCH
FOR A GERM-KILLER

It has often happened in the history of chemistry and medicine that a researcher in pursuit of one remedy has come up with something quite different. Such was the case with aspirin. The men who started the work that was to lead to the discovery of what would become the number one fever-fighter and painkiller were looking for a safe germ-killer.

It all began at the University of Leipzig about a hundred years ago. The German surgeon Carl Thiersch (1822-1895), who was made famous by a skin-graft procedure he introduced in 1874, brought a problem to his good friend Hermann Kolbe (1818-1884). He told the renowned chemist that he had been thinking for some time about treating patients internally with carbolic acid. Obviously, however, this acid was too dangerous for such use. Could Kolbe suggest a chemical he might substitute—a chemical that would slowly turn into carbolic acid inside the body?

The chemist replied that he knew just the thing. Twenty years earlier he had found a way to synthesize salicylic acid out of carbolic acid. He had discovered also that salicylic acid slowly breaks down in the test tube to make carbolic acid all over again. At the time he had not known to what use he might put his discovery. But now it was the obvious solution to Thiersch's problem.

The surgeon asked if Kolbe was certain that salicylic acid would turn back to carbolic acid in the body.

Kolbe was quite certain. After all, he pointed out, the body is nothing but a great test tube.

Kolbe and his assistants went to work. It was known that carbolic acid—phenol, as it is now called—killed germs. But as Thiersch had pointed out to Kolbe, it was too caustic to drink. Kolbe was convinced that salicylic acid would do the job safely as it slowly turned back into carbolic acid in the stomach.

Kolbe and his assistants were chemists. They knew little of the finer points of testing a germ-killer. But they produced quantities of salicylic acid and went to work with a will.

They tested it on meat in the process of decaying and on milk that was turning sour. They tried to kill both harmless yeasts and deadly microscopic germs taken from the bodies of dead men. They attempted to keep mold out of beer.

Ordinarily, milk went sour in three days. It stayed fresh for a week when salicylic acid was added. It was reasonable to assume that the salicylic acid turning into carbolic acid killed the microbes in the milk. If further proof were needed, salicylic acid was found to keep meat from decaying for a month and to prevent wine from turning sour.

The experimenting begun early in the winter of 1873 was wild and careless—even crazy. Kolbe would have condemned it as unscientific if it had been done by anyone else. But he was so set on proving his theory that he forgave himself the very excesses he would have condemned.

In the spring of 1874, Kolbe informed Thiersch that all was ready. *He had proved that salicylic acid killed microbes.* Thiersch lost no time in backing his friend's claim.

"Six days ago," he announced a week later, "I amputated the leg of a young fellow—just above the knee. I sprinkled salicylic acid on the stump and dressed it with bandages soaked in a solution of salicylic acid. Today we removed the dressing and found the wound entirely healed. [This salicylic acid] is so much better than straight carbolic, even externally. It causes so little irritation and so little damage to the tissue. . . ."[1]

Within weeks, salicylic acid was internationally famous. Doctors everywhere were reporting that it worked miraculously. They were so enthusiastic that they failed to recognize that the claims made for salicylic acid were wrong on two counts.

Kolbe's assertion that salicylic acid broke down in the body to form carbolic acid was in error. *If* salicylic acid was a germ-killer, it was a germ-killer in its own right.

The "miraculous cures" were not actually occurring as frequently as the enthusiasts were leading their colleagues to believe. There was always an excuse for failure.

A patient died from an infected wound that had been sprinkled with salicylic acid. His doctor concluded that he had not used enough of the powder.

A patient died from typhoid fever (or typhus or pneumonia) after he had been pumped full of salicylic acid. His doctor announced that treatment had been started too late.

A patient being treated internally with salicylic acid complained of a ringing or buzzing in his ears. Obviously he had been given too large a dose.

The believers insisted that it was all a matter of determining right dosages. Once they licked this problem, salicylic acid would be the answer to all infections.

A year went by. The doubters began to outnumber the enthusiasts. They admitted that salicylic acid undoubtedly made their patients feel better, but they were beginning to find that it only *cured* patients who would have lived anyway.

The fact was that patients were dying from the "killer" diseases in as great numbers as previously. It was true that when salicylic acid was given to weak, sick, feverish typhoid patients, their fever dropped within a few hours and they felt like living again. Nonetheless they died a few days later. Patients with typhus, pneumonia, and other like diseases reacted in exactly the same way.

SALICYLIC ACID
REDUCES FEVER

Carl Emil Buss, a young doctor working at a hospital in St. Gallen, Switzerland, was considerably bothered by the difference between what his chiefs told him salicylic acid should do and his own experience with it.

First, there was the old woman with typhoid fever. She had been given salicylic acid for fourteen days. Each day, within two hours of taking the dose, her temperature dropped and she felt more comfortable. She died on the fifteenth day.

Second, a young man with pneumonia and high fever had been given salicylic acid three times. Each time his temperature dropped, but he nevertheless died.

Third, salicylic acid brought down the temperature of an old man with painful rheumatic joints and high fever, and he was able to go home. True, he did not die; but then, Dr. Buss reminded himself, nobody died of rheumatism.

Reflecting on these three recent cases, Dr. Buss saw the common denominator.

The temperature of a feverish patient always goes down when he is given salicylic acid.

The fever might come back, but another dose of salicylic acid would bring it down again. The patient might ultimately live or die, but a dose of salicylic acid was always followed by reduced fever.

All very fine, but salicylic acid was not supposed to be a fever cure. That, Dr. Buss had been taught, was the job of quinine—or such hard-to-use drugs as veratrine, aconite, willow bark. . . .

Dr. Buss's thinking came to an abrupt halt. He had read somewhere that natives had used willow bark as a remedy for centuries. Could there be more than superstition to this folk-practice? He turned to his books to see what he might find. The botanical name of the white willow is *Salix alba*. . . . *Salix*—salicylic acid.

Then he remembered something else. Oil of wintergreen was a plant remedy long recognized in the relief of fevers and of rheumatic pain. Oil of wintergreen contained methyl salicylate.

Dr. Buss did not permit himself to be carried away by what he had found. He systematically tested his theory on scores of patients. Finally he was satisfied. He prepared a scientific paper in which he concluded: "Salicylic acid has, in my hands, invariably reduced fevers. . . . The cause of the fever is not important."[2]

Overnight this unknown researcher became world-famous.

A REMEDY
FOR RHEUMATISM

But Carl Buss was just one man and a young one at that. The time had come for others to settle once and for all what salicylic acid would and would not do.

Dr. Carl Anton Ewald of Berlin had tried salicylic acid in all his typhoid fever cases. He reported with some disappointment that his deaths from typhoid were as numerous as in former years, perhaps more so. No one disputed his claim that salicylic acid was no cure for typhoid. But his colleagues reminded him that it certainly reduced dangerous temperatures.

On the other side of the coin, Dr. Franz Stricker, also of Berlin, found that rheumatic patients treated with salicylic acid not only experienced a drop in fever but also much relief of the pain of rheumatism. "After two days of treatment, the swollen joints went back to normal, the reddening disappeared, and the pain stopped," he announced. "I have tried salicylic acid on all types of rheumatism, and I have noted always the same results. I even notice the same relief when my patients have the rheumatic pains with no fever at all. Undoubtedly, salicylic acid is a specific against rheumatism!"[3]

Once Dr. Stricker had revealed that salicylic acid stopped the pain of rheumatism, other doctors found that it also stopped the pain of neuralgia, sciatica, neuritis, and headache.

Hermann Kolbe had gone hunting for a germ-killer and was convinced he had found it. Instead he lighted the path to an unsurpassed fever-fighter and painkiller.

KNORR ACCIDENTALLY PRODUCES ANTIPYRINE

Kolbe's was not the only error in the aspirin story. Twenty-four-year-old Ludwig Knorr (1859-1921) of the University of Würzburg was responsible for the second.

Now that an effective antidote to fever, rheumatism, and pain had been discovered, scientists inevitably began searching for something better.

Quinine had been the standard remedy in fever cases up to this point. Salicylic acid was proving itself as effective and was certainly less costly to produce. Furthermore, it was then the only known treatment for rheumatism. Morphine was a more potent painkiller, but salicylic acid was a much safer drug in the relief of modern pain.

But the scientists remained convinced that there must be something still more wonderful just over the horizon.

Quinine offered an obvious point for investigation. After all, it was a long recognized fever-killer. German chemists went to work to find out what part of the quinine molecule controlled fever. They were quick to abandon the few quinine derivatives they uncovered. All of them caused chills, turned the skin blue, and disrupted the kidneys.

However, in 1833, ten years after Kolbe went to work on his would-be germ-killer, young Ludwig Knorr was still investigating the quinine molecule. His approach was different from that of researchers who had preceded him. They had taken quinine apart and studied its components. Knorr decided to take basic chemicals, put them together, and produce "something like quinine."

His choice fell on a mixture of methyl-phenyl-hydrazine and ethyl-aceto-acetate. The result was white crystals soluble in water and alcohol.

He had his product, but how to test it? At the University of Erlangen, fifty miles distant, he had studied under a Dr. Wilhelm Filehne, an authority on fever and fever drugs. He now wrote his former professor, telling him that he had "recently synthesized in my laboratory a new compound which is undoubtedly some kind of quinine derivative. Could you do me the great kindness to test this and give me the benefit of your experience and great knowledge."[4]

Just another quinine derivative, thought Dr. Filehne, who had tested so many promising ones to no purpose. But the following week he had a few hours open, so he decided to comply with his former student's request.

What he found surprised him. He did not stop when the few hours he had assigned were spent. He put Knorr's crystals through every possible laboratory test and proved in the hospital that they were safe to use. Knorr's new chemical did not cure malarial fever for which quinine was specific. But it worked like a charm on fevers associated with pneumonia, tuberculosis, erysipelas, typhoid, and typhus.

Filehne reported to his "dear young friend" that he didn't know what his product was but "as an antifever drug it is one of the most remarkable I have ever seen." He suggested that Knorr name it *antipyrine* from the Greek word for fever—*pyretos*.[5]

German doctors gave antipyrine to rheumatic patients and watched it bring relief to aching, swollen joints. They used it for headache, backache, and neuralgia with invariable success. Glowing reports were pouring in to Dr. Knorr.

It was only then that he became aware that he had been guilty of error. He had not produced synthetic quinine as he had set out to do. Careful chemical testing now revealed that methyl-phenyl-hydrazine and ethyl-aceto-acetate did not react on each other as he had supposed they would. He had actually created a brand-new compound of a type never seen before. It was a totally artificial drug that existed nowhere in the world outside of a laboratory.

Thanks to his error, Ludwig Knorr had produced the first great completely synthetic drug. At the same time, he had laid the foundations for a great industry—the synthetic drug industry.

The Germans went quickly to the forefront in this new field. They discovered that the raw materials used in their already flourishing dye industry were the raw materials of synthetic drugs. Dye works were easily converted into drug factories. With this built-in lead, Germany was to enjoy a forty-year monopoly of synthetic drugs.

ANOTHER
ACCIDENTAL DISCOVERY

With the first two great fever-fighters and painkillers—salicylic acid and antipyrine—discovered by chance, it is hard to believe that there could be a third such discovery in the same area of investigation. Yet that is just what happened.

In 1886, three years after Knorr developed antipyrine, Dr. Adolf Kussmaul (1822-1902) and his associates at a small clinic in the Alsace town of Strasbourg were seeking new information on the stomach and the digestive tract. Dr. Arnold Cahn was

working on the acids of the stomach. Dr. Paul Hepp was looking for a cure for trichinosis, a disease caused by eating raw or
insufficiently cooked pork. Neither was pleased when Dr. Kussmaul assigned them a new job. He showed them a nasty worm
that got into a patient's stomach and burrowed into the intestinal
wall. He proposed that they find a chemical that would kill it
without harming the patient.

Cahn and Hepp decided that they would first try naphthalene,
the substance of which mothballs are now made. They requested
a supply from the storekeeper.

He told them that the bottle recently in use was empty. However, he had an unopened bottle which he was sure was naphthalene. Unfortunately, the label had had liquid spilt on it and could
not be read.

The contents certainly looked like naphthalene. That seems to
have been enough for Cahn and Hepp, who were eager to get
this worm business over with and get back to their interrupted
investigations. A week later they were still trying to kill worms
with what they had supposed was naphthalene.

Dr. Hepp had had enough. He grabbed the bottle and announced that he was going to see if the stuff would cure anything.

He had a patient whose bowels were crammed with everything
in the textbook. He gave him a dose of the white powder. A few
hours later he was back with Cahn blurting out that naphthalene
reduces fever.

Cahn retorted that this was impossible—that someone in Berlin
had tried it and it didn't work.

Hepp was unmoved. That morning his patient's temperature
was five degrees above normal. Thirty minutes after a dose of
this naphthalene it was down to normal.

Cahn grabbed the bottle, opened it, and sniffed. There was no
odor. Obviously it was not naphthalene.

How these two young doctors had managed to work with this

chemical for a week without noticing the absence of the distinctive smell of mothballs remains a mystery.

Hepp proposed that they ask his cousin at the dye factory to analyze the substance and tell them what it actually was.

Dr. Hepp of the Biebach Dye Works had no difficulty in identifying his cousin's white powder. It was a substance long known to chemists—acetanilid, a combination of acetic acid and aniline. Aniline is used in the manufacture of dyes.

The two Strasbourg physicians tested their newfound antipyretic on animals. It worked in every case. Then they tried it on a couple of dozen patients with equal success.

In reporting their discovery to the medical community, they named their new antipyretic *antifebrin.*

A PILE
OF WASTE

The fourth great fever-fighter was developed six months after the introduction of antifebrin. Its discovery was also accidental but in a somewhat different sense. If there had not been a storage problem at a dye factory, *phenacetin* might not have been developed.

Carl Duisburg was director of research at the Friedrich Bayer and Company dye works. He was faced with about fifty tons of yellowish powder that had accumulated in the courtyard. It was a useless by-product of dye production—crude para-amino-phenol.

Duisburg had to choose between paying to have this waste hauled away and converting it into something that could be sold. He decided on the latter course.

He looked up the formula for para-amino-phenol. Then on a

hunch he compared it with antifebrin. He found the formulas were not very different and concluded that, if the amine group were acetylated, something practical might result.

The job turned out simpler than he had any right to expect. Soon small quantities of his new product were being tested on patients in the Freiburg hospital. The tests were highly successful. The accumulation of yellow powder was carefully removed from the courtyard and processed into this new, safe, effective fever-fighter. Phenacetin enjoyed an advantage over its older relatives. It was inexpensive to produce because it was made from a by-product.

Carl Duisburg was highly praised for his ingenuity but he did his best to duck the compliments, insisting that it was part of his job to turn waste products into something that could be sold. Nevertheless, he was later to head the I. G. Farbenindustrie dye and drug trust.

In fact, *turn waste products into something that could be sold* became part of the basic philosophy of German industrial chemistry.

Phenacetin was the first antipyretic that was not accidentally discovered during a search for something else. It was scientifically planned and did just what was expected of it. It was followed by *aminopyrine,* also called *pyramidon,* which was Knorr's antipyrine with a few flourishes added. Aminopyrine was actually superior to antipyrine in that it was effective in smaller doses that had a longer-lasting effect.

Cinchophen was sixth in line. Cinchophen had the advantage of also being effective in gout, but it is seldom used today because it frequently produces serious side effects, including a fatal form of hepatitis.

Then as the nineteenth century reached its end, the stage was set for number seven.

HOFFMAN
NAMES ASPIRIN

About the time Hermann Kolbe first synthesized salicylic acid from carbolic acid back in 1853, another German prepared a derivative of this new chemical. He described acetyl-salicylic acid and then set it aside as worthless. For almost fifty years acetyl-salicylic acid was no more than a name in the textbooks.

In 1899, Felix Hoffman (1868-1946), a staff chemist at Bayer and Company, found himself under pressure from two sources.

His bosses ordered him to find a fever-fighter superior to salicylic acid.

His rheumatic father, who was taking salicylic acid constantly, complained about the vile pills that burned his throat and made him vomit.

Felix shut himself up in his laboratory and worked his way through all the potential fever-killers. He was a patient, painstaking man. It was inevitable that he should finally come to acetyl-salicylic acid. He turned it over for testing to Dr. Heinrich Dreser, head of the Bayer research department.

Acetyl-salicylic acid passed its tests with flying colors. Dreser and Hoffman congratulated each other on their success. Dreser, however, had one reservation. He didn't like the name of the new drug. Acetyl-salicylic acid was just too complicated and too long.

They considered cutting "acetyl" to "a" and calling it "a-salicylic" or "a-salicin" and then decided to try and get away altogether from the word salicylic. Some people fought shy of it. Felix Hoffman's father was a good example.

They had, of course, always thought of the bark of the willow —and *Salix*—as nature's source of salicylic acid. But about sixty years earlier someone had found salicylic acid in *Spiraea* plants. Hoffman now remembered this. He proposed calling their new drug "acetyl-spiric acid" or, perhaps, "a-spirin."

It was not too great a mental jump from *a-spirin* to *aspirin*.

Aspirin has proved invaluable in checking the pains and fevers of everyday life, but there is one form of pain that it barely touches, an inflammation of the joints—usually the great toe—known as gout.

Fortunately, a plant remedy for gout has been known for thirty-five centuries, although its full medical acceptance did not come until about two hundred years ago.

Five

Calming

a Swollen Toe ❧❧

⌐ *Colchicine*

COLCHICUM
THE POISON

Colchicine is an alkaloid obtained from the seeds and bulbous root (the corm) of the *Colchicum autumnale* or meadow saffron. This member of the lily family is also known as the autumn crocus because, while the leaves appear in the spring, it does not flower until fall. The corms of the *Colchicum autumnale* are not alone in yielding colchicine. However, they are the most productive, and the corms of some species offer no colchicine at all.

Colchicum rivals opium for the honor of being the oldest plant remedy still in use. Both are mentioned in the Ebers papyrus, the Egyptian record dating back to the sixteenth century B.C.

Colchicum's major claim to medical fame has been as a remedy for gouty arthritis, a painful affliction of a single joint, frequently the great toe. But colchicum's history has been checkered. This is largely because colchicum is a deadly poison. When used for medical purposes, it must be given in small, carefully controlled doses.

Colchicum's use as a poison dates back as far as Greek legend. The sorceress Medea, whose story is told in a play by Euripides and an opera by Cherubini, helped Jason obtain the Golden Fleece. Medea was a bloodthirsty opportunist. She killed her brother in order to slow her father's pursuit when she was running away with Jason. She killed her two sons to spite Jason who had deserted her. She also killed the daughter of King Creon, whom Jason had set in her place. Incidentally, she killed King Creon of Corinth himself.

These final murders were brought about through the instrument of a robe that Medea had sent as a gift to the Corinthian princess. The robe was soaked in extract of colchicum. The story goes that King Creon and his daughter died as soon as they touched the poisoned robe.

Moving to historic times, around A.D. 77 Pedanios Dioskorides wrote a book describing the preparation, storage, genuineness, use, doses, and effects of simple drugs derived from six hundred plants. He dismissed colchicum as a deadly poison with which slaves would often end their lives.

By medieval times, such recognition as had been given colchicum's medicinal value was outweighed by its reputation as a poison. The Abbess Hildegard (1099-1179) of Bingen, whose word was as good as law throughout Germany, forbade its use. She described it as a deadly poison and not a health-giving drug.

William Turner is regarded as the English father of scientific botany. In 1548, he advised against the use of colchicum. He was supported by the scholarly Elizabethan physician William Bullein who wrote in 1579, "It is well that [colchicum] be not used." Apothecary John Gerard said in 1597 that colchicum "can be very hurtful to the stomach."[1]

Colchicum was listed in the first edition of the *London Pharmacopoeia* published in 1618, but was dropped from all editions appearing between 1650 and 1788. This was brought about by the influential Thomas Sydenham, who declared that all purgative treatments were bad because they bring on what they are meant to keep off. Up to that time, colchicum had been used as a purge. But advice from so great a medical authority as Sydenham was not to be lightly ignored. European physicians who were still using colchicum as a purgative in gout quickly abandoned the practice.

Meadow saffron grew wild in Herefordshire, England, as it did in the rich moist meadowlands of most of Europe. It had long been prized as a household remedy for gout and arthritis. When it lost favor with a medical profession that took to calling it "colchicum perniciosum," the Herefordshire farmers rooted it out as a "poisonous weed."

OTHER TREATMENT
FOR GOUT

There is no certainty when colchicum was first recognized as a treatment for gout. However, the best evidence points to around A.D. 550. Even then, its acceptance was far from universal, and most of those who had been using colchicum gave up the practice when the Abbess Hildegard prohibited its use in the twelfth century.

This was unfortunate. The remedies substituted for the relief of the pain of gout were usually worthless, frequently ridiculous, and sometimes frightening.

One fantastic remedy favored during the Middle Ages involved soaking the aching foot in a basin of fresh blood. This practice reached an extreme when Mathew d'Agello, Norman chancellor of Sicily, had Arab prisoners decapitated in order to provide fresh blood in which to soak his gouty toe.

An earlier and more humane approach dates back to Rome at the beginning of the Christian era. The Greek physician Antonius Musa is said to have cured both the Emperor Augustus Caesar and the poet Horace of gout by prescribing cold baths. It may be assumed that the shock of immersion in cold water neutralized the pain.

For the most part, the turn was to herbal remedies. The majority of these contained nothing that could be expected to relieve the pain of gout. An early British example involved a mixture of leek, pepper, cumin, and laurel berries. The Duke of Portland's

Gout Powder, which appeared on the market in the middle of the eighteenth century, was a combination of birthwort root, gentian root, leaves of germander, ground pine, and centaury.

A popular antidote to gout involved charm necklaces and bracelets worn about the wrist, the arm, and even the leg. Such superstitious practices might have been expected of the ignorant peasantry but they actually ran through all levels of society. No less a person than Queen Elizabeth I's lord treasurer, William Cecil, Lord Burleigh, always wore an amulet around his leg. It was a blue ribbon studded with small shells. He was firmly convinced that it protected him from gout.

While colchicum was highly suspect as a medicine to be taken internally, it was nonetheless associated with gout in the minds of many. This made it a natural for those who believed in good-luck pieces. A colchicum corm might be carried in the pocket. Roots of colchicum might be strung together and worn as a necklace. This practice even spread to the army. On one occasion a British officer was asked by a superior why his uniform was in such disorder. He explained that he was wearing a colchicum necklace beneath his tunic. The Bavarian Leonhard Fuchs (1501-1566), professor of medicine at the University of Tübingen, published a history of plants in 1542. He said of colchicum as a gout preventive that, worn as a necklace, it has the added advantage of killing fleas on the wearer's person.

A Far Eastern approach to the treatment of gout was slightly more scientific. It involved burning small capsules of herbs known as *moxa* or Chinese wormwood on the skin of patients. This process must have been extremely painful and, in light of modern knowledge, it can have served at best as a counterirritant. However, it can be regarded as no more inhuman than such Western practices as bloodletting and the raising of blisters under the pretext of drawing poison from the body. One may scoff at the crudity of such remedies, but their principles are followed to this day in the unpleasant plasters and medicated pads that are sold to the gullible to draw out the poison. The best that can be said for the modern version is that it is irritating rather than painful.

When Thomas Sydenham condemned all purgative treatments, including colchicum for gout, he did himself a great disservice. He suffered from gout for thirty years, so severely in fact that he had finally to quit the practice of medicine because of the pain.

Sydenham subscribed to the popular view that gout was an affliction of the aristocrat and the bon vivant. Gout, he wrote in 1682, "destroys more rich men than poor persons, and more wise men than fools. . . ."[2]

His conclusion is only partially valid. Gout results from an accumulation of uric acid crystals in a joint, frequently the great toe. The accumulated crystals are responsible for the extreme pain, and even deformity, symptomatic of gout. Uric acid crystals form when the body chemistry balance is disturbed. Such imbalance is caused by the consumption of certain foods.

In former times, the foods in question were available to the limited few who could afford them. This supported the assumption that gout was a rich man's disease. But today these foods are common in the diets of many people. We can all get gout. Still another factor is involved. There can be a predisposition to the disturbance in body chemistry that causes the formation of uric acid crystals. Such predisposition can be transmitted from parent to offspring. Consequently, there is some justification for regarding gout as a hereditary disease.

Sydenham was scornful of self-indulgent gout victims who sat before the fire with the painful foot on a hassock. He referred to this practice as the sweat cure before the fire. Instead, he advocated fresh air, keeping the mind quiet, and long horseback rides. He also favored small beer before dinner.

The fate of the gout sufferer was not improved a century later when the Scotsman William Cullen declared gout to be an affliction of the nervous system. With no proven cure to offer, Cullen tried everything in the book. His program included bodily exercise, abstinence from animal food and fermented liquors, blood-letting, the use of agents to relieve inflammation, blistering, Peruvian bark, Portland powder (birthwort and gentian), and sleep-inducing drugs.

The fact that gout was the result of an excess of uric acid had been known to physicians for some time. Doctors followed the practice of tightly binding the foot in an attempt to keep the uric acid out of the patient's great toe. Then, toward the middle of the nineteenth century it was discovered in the laboratory that lithium would dissolve uric acid. The doctors at last had a remedy.

At about the time of this discovery, gout victims began going to mineral spring resorts (spas) in continental Europe to "take the waters." Analysis revealed that the mineral water of spas popular for gouty conditions had a high lithium content. Today we use a pure synthetic, benemid (probenecid), rather than lithium to reduce the uric acid level in patients with gouty arthritis.

At this point an important distinction must be made. Neither benemid nor lithium *relieves the pain* of acute attacks of gout. This is the province of colchicum and its alkaloid derivative colchicine. At the same time, neither colchicum nor colchicine does anything to reduce the buildup of uric acid in the patient's system. This is the province of benemid.

COLCHICUM
AS A MEDICINE

In the beginning colchicum was considered a poison. Because it was condemned by many physicians, unfortunate substitutes were often employed in the treatment of gout. Colchicum nonetheless has had a long history as a medicine.

With the fall of Rome, the world center of the arts and sciences shifted to Constantinople. It was here in the Byzantine Empire that colchicum was first used as a remedy for gout.

Hippocrates is believed to have been the first to describe gout in man, although there are earlier descriptions of a similar affliction of the joints of beasts of burden.

The disease was originally called *podagra,* from the Greek words *pous* meaning foot and *agra* meaning seizure. In fact, podagra remained the name of the disease until the thirteenth century A.D.

Hippocrates's remedy for podagra was a purge made from white hellebore. White hellebore is a botanical cousin of the colchicum family.

Colchicum itself was regarded by the ancient Greeks as a powerful purgative, but there is little reason to suppose that they thought of it particularly as a remedy for gout. Indeed, it is questionable whether the Greeks, including Hippocrates, thought of gout as anything more than one manifestation of arthritis. Podagra was arthritis settling in the foot just as cheiragra was arthritis of the hand, pechyagra of the elbow, gonagra of the knee, and so on.

The first person clearly to recognize gout as a distinct entity was the Roman doctor Caelius Aurelianus writing around A.D. 500. He pointed out the bony involvement that could lead to deformity and described a sensation of ants crawling over the part.

Alexander (526-605) of Tralles was a Byzantine Christian physician. Judging by his own writings and those of others since his time, he established colchicum as a specific remedy for gout. He distinguished gout from arthritis in general on the basis that colchicum was effective in the treatment of gout but not of other forms of arthritis. Therefore, he argued, there were many variations of arthritic disease, each of which might require a remedy of its own.

Alexander obtained his colchicum from the corm of *Colchicum variegatum,* a species of crocus larger but less effective than *Colchicum autumnale.* Still, he was very much impressed by the efficacy of his preparation. He told of relief from pain and reduction of swelling in the joint within a matter of hours.

However, his fellow Byzantine Aetios (502-575), of Amida, counseled caution. He agreed with Alexander that colchicum rapidly calms pain, generally within two days, permitting the sufferer to resume his usual occupation. But he warned that some, in the agony of gout, took too large a dose of colchicum. This, he said, was bad for the stomach, producing nausea and loss of appetite. Aetios admitted that these side effects could sometimes be reduced by the addition of certain aromatic spices. Still, he advised against the use of colchicum except "in the case of those who are pressed for time by urgent affairs of business. . . ."[3]

Physicians of the Moslem Empire leaned toward spices, herbs, and plant life generally as a source of medicines. They made a careful study of colchicum and it is found included in a pharmacopoeia written by Abu Mansur Muwaffak bin Ali al-Harawi in A.D. 968. Moslem caliphs used colchicum for the relief of gout up to the eighteenth century.

The first European medical school was founded at Salerno near Naples in 1075. By this time the virtue of colchicum for the treatment of gout was so well established that this therapy was taught at the school. However, within a hundred years colchicum had fallen into disrepute.

A contributing factor may have been the difficulty of obtaining the right corms and then properly treating them. The Salerno medical school used a textbook known as the *Antidotarium,* a compilation of remedies in common use. It was corrected and enlarged in the middle of the twelfth century by Nicholas Salernitanus (*ca.* 1140). Nicholas said that corms must be gathered in the spring and dried a short time in the sun. Then they must be hung in the dark at an even temperature for at least six months. Their coverings must not be damaged in any way in the process.

If the producer failed to observe all these requirements, the colchicum would lose its potency. In addition, as we have seen, only the corms of certain colchicum species produce the drug.

Colchicum was not entirely dropped from medieval medical practice. It was touted by itinerant herbalists. It was used by doctors catering to the gouty upper class. Such physicians had learned colchicum's virtues, and probably its limitations, from practical experience.

Among them was another noted Salernitan, Gilbertus Anglicus (*ca.* 1250), who produced a compendium of the works of all medical writers to date. It has been described as "a pretty good medical library for a practitioner in the thirteenth century."[4] Gilbertus named the colchicum preparation that he used *Cothopcie Alexanderine* in honor of the discoverer of the remedy, Alexander of Tralles.

In 1282 the physician to the Byzantine Emperor Paleologus VIII wrote his master a prescription that involved a small, safe quantity of colchicum combined with a large dose of aloes. The good doctor does not seem to have had much confidence in his remedy because he leaned rather more heavily on divine intervention. "This will cure you," he told Paleologus, "provided we have the assistance of Heaven, the intercession of the Blessed Virgin Mother, and the help of God."[5] This appears to be the last recorded use of colchicum in medieval Europe.

But the botanists and herbalists never lost their faith in the medicinal properties of colchicum. The sixteenth century saw them again bringing it to the notice of physicians. The doctors now rejected it on entirely new grounds. They would not adopt anything approved of and used by the Moslems. Nonetheless, a few patients were relieved of pain by the inclusion of native-grown colchicum in the purgatives that were the traditional treatment for gout. Ambroise Paré (1509-1590), the famous French military surgeon, made use of colchicum. However, it must be recognized that this was merely one of a score of remedies, traditional, medical, and surgical, that he employed. His simple, over-riding motive was to get rid of the pain.

Colchicum was rescued from oblivion in 1763. Professor Baron Antony von Stoerk (1731-1803), head of the Medical Clinic in Vienna and physician to the Empress Maria Theresa, was the agent. He had studied under Hermann Boerhaave (1668-1738) whose writings and teaching brought fame to the Dutch University of Leyden. In 1725 Boerhaave developed gout. It had become so painful by 1729 that he had to abandon most of his teaching. He died nine years later. But even if von Stoerk had rehabilitated colchicum forty years sooner, it would not have helped his master. He used colchicum to treat dropsy, not gout.

Universal acceptance of colchicum in the treatment of gout did not come for another fifty years. Nonetheless, von Stoerk made a major contribution. He established that it was possible to take "small quantities of this deadly poison regularly without risking sudden death, and that the patient might even benefit from such temerity."[6]

The revival of colchicum as a remedy for gout must be credited to Nicholas Husson, a French army officer.

A SECRET
REMEDY

Toward the end of the reign of Louis XV, Husson concocted a secret remedy which he called *Eau médicinale d'Husson*. This "quack" remedy was an instant success with gout victims. A two-dose bottle sold for the equivalent of $5. Husson advertised his tonic as a cure for all ills. This led to its being banned by the Paris police in 1778. But the prohibition was lifted after four days, seemingly at the insistence of the gout sufferers. The basic ingredient in Eau médicinale was extract of *Colchicum autumnale*. However, this fact was not revealed until 1814.

Eau médicinale d'Husson was vehemently denounced by the medical profession because it was a patent medicine. But there were a few mavericks who were willing to investigate this remedy that gout sufferers praised so highly. One of them, Dr. Edwin Godden Jones, introduced Eau médicinale into England in 1808. Not only did he test the remedy exhaustively in his practice but in 1810 he wrote *An Account of the Remarkable Effects of the Eau médicinale d'Husson in the Gout.* He dedicated this book to Sir Walter Farquhar, who was then physician to the Prince Regent (later George IV). Sir Walter did not refuse the honor, but he nevertheless declined to test the secret formula on his royal patient.

In 1810, a few bottles of Eau médicinale came into the hands of Sir Joseph Banks, the respected president of the Royal Society. Sir Joseph tried the remedy and reported considerable success. This later inspired Sir Everard Home, generally an extremely conservative physician, to produce his own "wine" for the relief of gout. He cooked colchicum corms at a gentle heat in sherry wine for six days before bottling.

But it remained for Dr. James Want to establish that colchicum was the basic ingredient in the Husson creation. He produced a rival product and not only demonstrated its effectiveness in the treatment of forty patients but also showed it to be identical with what Husson was selling.

Want published his findings in 1814 in *The Medical and Physical Journal.* However, disclosure of his formula had little effect on Husson sales. The Frenchman had found a means of standardizing and preserving his product. He established an outlet at the corner of St. James Street, London, not long after Want's revelation.

In 1817, the Prince Regent was being treated for gout by Sir

Henry Halford and Sir John Knighton. He was taking 1,200 drops of laudanum daily without relief of pain. He announced to his physicians: "Gentlemen, I have taken your half-measures long enough to please you . . . From now on I shall take colchicum to please myself."[7] Thanks to colchicum, Louis XVIII of France, who had gone into retirement because of his severe gout, became well enough to return to the throne in 1815, after Napoleon's defeat.

Sydney Smith, the noted English essayist who died in 1845, was loud in his praise of colchicum. Seeing the autumn crocus in flower, he said, ". . . who would guess the virtue of that little plant? But I find the power of *colchicum* so great that if I feel a little gout coming on, I go into the garden and hold out my toe to that plant, and it gets well immediately."[8]

Led by Sir Charles Scudamore, nineteenth-century physicians enthusiastically adopted the use of colchicum. However, there were holdouts. An outstanding French consultant, Armand Trousseau, felt that the side effects of the unstandardized preparations then available were too serious to justify its use. Others admitted that colchicum relieved the pain of acute gout but believed that its use both aggravated the disease and increased the frequency of attacks.

However, these objections and difficulties were overcome by improved chemical techniques. In the same year in which they isolated quinine (1820) Pelletier and Caventou discovered the alkaloid colchicine. Sixty-four years later, Houdé produced colchicine in crystalline form. His crystals were stable, reliable, and easy to take in exact dosage.

COLCHICUM INTRODUCED
INTO AMERICA

Benjamin Franklin showered so many benefits on his country—as statesman, diplomat, philosopher, and inventor—that it would be nice to be able to credit him with one more: colchicum.

Maurice A. Schnitker, writing of Benjamin Franklin in 1936, refers to an "interesting legend to the effect that in one of his European travels he observed the use of the wine of colchicum in the treatment of gout; he tried it himself, and obtaining beneficial results, he purchased some which he sent back to America, advising it as a substitute for morphine. According to the story, he is thus given credit for introducing wine of colchicum into this country."[9]

This legend was generally accepted until twenty years ago. The suggestion that an American hero, sage, and savant introduced a useful drug to his country was hard to discredit.

Some set the date when Nicolas Husson produced his secret remedy for gout as late as 1780. This is clearly wrong, since its sale in Paris was briefly banned in 1778. There are even grounds for believing that the preparation appeared as early as 1770.

Benjamin Franklin suffered his first attack of gout in 1749. He was in France as U.S. representative from 1779 to 1785. He died in 1790. He therefore had ample opportunity to sample a few bottles of Eau médicinale d'Husson. He might have arranged to ship some to friends back home.

James Want did not identify colchicum as the active ingredient in Eau médicinale until twenty-four years after Franklin's death. Franklin may have taken colchicum without knowing it, but he certainly could not have introduced it into America as such.

Furthermore, there is plenty of evidence to suggest that Franklin would never have touched Husson's proprietary medicine. He was strongly opposed to all forms of quackery.

In 1767 he had written of William Pitt's gout: "It is said that his constitution is totally destroyed and gone, partly through his own quacking with it."[10] He was fond of quoting an Italian epitaph, "I was well, I would be better, I took physic and died."[11] Toward the end of his life he said: "Quacks are the greatest liars in the world, except their patients."[12] In 1784 he wrote to John Jay: "My stomach performs well its functions. The latter is very material to the preservation of health. I therefore take no drugs, lest I should disorder it."[13]

It seems most unlikely that, knowingly or unknowingly, Franklin himself took the drug colchicum or that he introduced it into the United States. Furthermore, Eau médicinale did not cross the English Channel until 1808. It is highly improbable that it made an earlier crossing of the Atlantic Ocean.

This assumption is borne out by the fact that as late as 1812 the *New England Journal of Medicine and Surgery* published an English suggestion that Eau médicinale was "a mixture of three parts of wine of white hellebore to one of wine of opium."[14] The following year the *Journal* recommended Eau médicinale in the treatment of gout on the basis of English experience, but it did not reveal until 1815 Want's determination that the basic ingredient in Husson's remedy was colchicum.

The first official *Pharmacopoeia of the United States,* published in 1820, included methods of preparing wine of colchicum and syrup of colchicum. This was the year in which Pelletier and Caventou isolated colchicine.

Thirty years after Franklin's death, colchicum and colchicine had arrived in the United States to stay.

HANDLE
WITH CARE

Colchicine is unquestionably an irritant that must be handled with care. It must be given at the first indication of an oncoming attack if it is to be effective in relieving the pain of gouty arthritis. Properly used, it counteracts the pain of gout. But to this day *nobody knows why.*

A similar lack of knowledge is evident in the use of digitalis and other drugs. These fascinating gaps are among the elements that make medicine and the related sciences an intriguing field for people with inquiring minds and character enough to persist through a long investigation. Many important discoveries have still to be made in medicine. Medical research remains a wide-open and challenging line of work.

As new ideas are formulated, they are immediately publicized by the various news media. Thus, the effects of smoking the leaves of the nicotine plant is scarcely news today. What may be news to many is the medical use of another leaf—that of the purple foxglove.

The hearts of thousands of men and women who would otherwise be incapacitated or dead are kept going by this leaf.

Six

A Cure
for Dropsy
⌐ Digitalis

A SIMPLE
COUNTRY REMEDY

Dropsy is a condition in which the tissues and the cavities of the body fill up with water. One cause is failure of the heart muscles to contract forcefully enough to drive the blood through the circulatory system and back to the heart. This allows fluid to collect in the lungs, liver, legs, and abdomen. However, dropsy occurs so infrequently today that most people have never seen a case of it and may not even have heard the name.

Yet for thousands of years dropsy was one of the chief causes of death, and there was little that the medical man could do about it. The patient simply became more and more bloated until finally he might be said to have drowned in his own body juices.

The farmers and housewives and their families fared better than the rich because they had little or no contact with doctors. For centuries a tall plant with long pointed leaves and purple bell-like flowers had grown wild throughout most of Europe. Wherever it grew, the simple country folk dried the heavy leaves and powdered them. They found that this powder brought relief to those among them suffering from dropsy.

The plant was the purple foxglove or *Digitalis purpurea*.

HOW FOXGLOVE
GOT ITS NAME

There are two accounts of how foxglove got its name.

The first suggests that it came from *folk glove*. "Folk" refers

129

to the "little folk" or fairies. This is supported by the fact that the Welsh word for foxglove is *menygellydon,* which means "elves' gloves."

The second version has it that the word comes from the Anglo-Saxon *foxes-glew* or "fox music." Reference here is to an ancient musical instrument that consisted of bells hung from an arched support. It is easy to see that the bell-shaped flowers hanging from the foxglove stalk could have reminded our ancestors of this instrument. This explanation is supported by the fact that the Norwegian word for foxglove, *revlecka,* also means "fox music."

Nor is the reason for the choice of *Digitalis* as the botanical family name any more certain. It is generally accepted that *Digitalis* comes from *digitus,* the Latin word for finger, selected because the tall, vertical stalk from which the foxglove flowers hang looks like a finger. However, the sixteenth-century botanist-physician Leonhard Fuchs, who is credited with naming *Digitalis,* is said to have taken it from the German name for the plant, *fingerhut,* which means "thimble" and refers to the bell-shaped flowers of the plant.

But whether foxglove got its name from the fairies or from music and digitalis refers to a finger or a thimble, the plant was used in England as a household remedy as far back as the tenth century A.D. At that early date, foxglove was being touted as a cure for epilepsy and the Italians were including it in a variety of quack healing ointments. By the thirteenth century, the Welsh "Physicians of Myddvai" were using foxglove as an external medicine.

HISTORY
OF FOXGLOVE

Foxglove's official medical history begins early in the sixteenth century.

In 1526, Peter Treveris published his *Great Herbal*. This book included an illustration of a plant resembling foxglove. It was recommended for "feebleness of the heart."[1] However, recent investigations suggest that the plant Treveris was discussing was probably not foxglove.

So credit for discovering the purple foxglove and naming it *Digitalis purpurea* goes to Leonhard Fuchs. Fuchs included digitalis as a purging and vomit-inducing medicine in his 1542 history of plants. He stated that the "plant is usually very effective in its action to thin, to dry up, to purge, and to free of obstructions."[2] This has been interpreted to mean that digitalis could be used to "scatter the dropsy."

A number of physicians who read Fuchs's book wrote him off as a mere flower-picker. Nor did they listen to John Gerard who observed in 1597 that, although foxglove had had no place in the medicine of the ancients, he had used it to produce vomiting. Then the Dutch medical biologist Rembert Dodoens (1517-1585) wrote that "for those who have water in the belly . . . it draws off the watery fluid, purifies the choleric fluid, and opens the obstruction."[3] He too was ignored.

Arezzo in Italy was the birthplace of Andrea Cesalpino (1519-1603). On the wall of a small house in this little Tuscan town there is an inscription that reads: "Here lived Andrea Cesalpino, discoverer of the circulation of the blood and first author of the classification of plants."[4]

The English physician William Harvey is generally recognized as the discoverer of the circulation of the blood. He introduced the concept in lectures before the Royal College of Physicians in about 1619. However, Cesalpino, professor of medicine at Pisa and physician to Pope Clement VIII, is credited by the Italians with making the discovery between 1571 and 1593.

The claim is a dubious one. Although Cesalpino seemed in some passages to refer to a general circulation of the blood, his ideas were quite vague, were not supported by convincing experiments, and had no influence on his Galenist contemporaries.[5]

Cesalpino also served as professor of botany and curator of the botanical gardens at Pisa. He recommended digitalis for use in dropsy cases but seems to have influenced few, if any, in its favor.

By 1661 digitalis had found its way into the *London Pharmacopoeia*. It was recommended for epilepsy and as a sedative. However, it remained for William Salmon (*ca.* 1690), an English physician-herbalist with a reputation for being conservative in the claims he made, to become the real champion of digitalis. This was in 1722.

Salmon sponsored digitalis as a cure for many major afflictions, including tuberculosis. Many of his claims for digitalis were actually in error, but his enthusiasm brought doctors who had previously ignored it under the foxglove banner.

Salmon can be pardoned for believing that digitalis cured tuberculosis. It was hard in his day to distinguish between dropsy of the chest, which digitalis does cure, and tuberculosis, which it definitely does not. In fact, this confusion between tuberculosis and dropsy was to plague doctors for another couple of hundred years. Furthermore, heart failure frequently affects the lungs. It was easy for eighteenth-century physicians to believe they were facing tuberculosis when they were actually dealing with heart failure, which is responsive to digitalis, and therefore, to believe that digitalis cured tuberculosis.

Whatever his mistakes, Salmon was quite clear in recommending digitalis as a cure for dropsy.

He was also very specific in his warnings that there could be violent reactions if digitalis were given in large doses. Unfortunately his recommendation of small doses was generally ignored. Consequently, the poisonous aspect of digitalis was emphasized. The situation was not helped when Holland's Hermann Boerhaave, "the general teacher of Europe," declared the drug to be a poison and cautioned against its use.

Then, to cap it all, in 1748 a Dr. Salerne of Orleans, seventy-five miles south of Paris, conducted an unfortunate experiment that was given wide publicity.

He had heard that a turkey had died after eating foxglove leaves. Deciding to investigate for himself, he forced foxglove leaves down the throats of two healthy turkeys until they could take no more. They died a few days later. An autopsy revealed that their intestines were shrunken and dry, looking as if they had been squeezed out like a sponge. It is obvious that these healthy turkeys had been violently subjected to the process by which water is squeezed out of bloated dropsy patients. All Dr. Salerne had proved was that an overdose of digitalis can prove fatal. However, he reported to the French Academy of Sciences that digitalis was a deadly poison. The Academy was at that time the final authority in European medicine. Salerne was in effect publishing his condemnation to the Western world. Digitalis was back on the black list. But the ignorant peasants, farmers, and old wives never heard of Dr. Salerne and his massacre of the turkeys. They went right on using digitalis as they had before Salmon.

This was fortunate. But for an old wives' tale, William Withering might not have introduced digitalis to the world of medicine a quarter of a century later nor written *An Account of the Foxglove, and Some of Its Medical Uses, with Practical Remarks on Dropsy, and Other Diseases* which appeared in 1785.

WILLIAM WITHERING
HEARS AN
OLD WIVES' TALE

William Withering (1741-1799) was born in the English village of Wellington in Shropshire, not far from Birmingham. His father, his grandfather, and two uncles were doctors. It was inevitable that young William would wind up in medical school.

At the University of Edinburgh, from which he obtained his medical degree in 1766, he excelled in medicine, surgery, anatomy, and chemistry, but did not like botany. At the age of twenty-three, he had spoken of "the disagreeable ideas I have formed of the study of botany."[6]

Ironically, Withering was to become one of the greatest medical botanists of all time. In 1766 he published *A Botanical Arrangement of All the Vegetables Naturally Grown in Great Britain According to the System of the Celebrated Linnaeus,* the first complete text on the plants of the British Isles to be written in English.

Withering was cautious in his approach. This caution is well illustrated by the fact that by the time his book was published he had already spent a year studying foxglove. Yet he made only one comment on its medicinal properties: "A dram of it taken inwardly excites violent vomiting. It is certainly a very active medicine and merits more attention than modern practice bestows on it."[7]

The change that occurred between 1764 and 1776 in Withering's attitude toward botany was prompted by two factors. First, his original practice was not a busy one. This left him plenty of time for outside pursuits. Secondly, he had a charming young patient named Helena Cooke whom he found it necessary to see almost daily. Miss Cooke passed the hours of her convalescence painting flowers. Dr. Withering fell into the habit of bringing her a different wildflower at each visit. This taught him the names of the various flowers, when they grew, where they grew, and how they grew. Five years of flower discussion with his patient led to marriage.

This alone would not have led to the intensive study of foxglove that was to make Withering famous. He was prompted by a patient who asked his advice concerning a secret family recipe for the cure of dropsy used by an old woman of Shropshire.

Dr. Withering told the patient that his medical training and experience had made it clear that there was no such thing as a cure for dropsy. The patient replied that she was sure Dr. Withering was right but added that it was surprising how many dropsy sufferers whom the doctors had given up had subsequently been cured by these herbs.

Faced with little alternative, Withering undertook to study the recipe. The list, he found, included about twenty herbs. He considered them one by one.

Primrose leaves, pondweed, hornwort, waxberries, ribwort—all useless. Wintergreen—just for flavoring. Foxglove. . . .

Foxglove—digitalis—a member of the same plant family as nicotine and belladonna. It was worth a try.

WITHERING WRITES
AN ACCOUNT OF FOXGLOVE

About this time Withering moved to Birmingham where he founded a clinic for the poor in which he treated some three thousand patients a year. Many of them were full of water and dying from dropsy. Foxglove might help them.

The question was how much to give them. He tried a few grains on one patient and the water poured out. Another needed twice as much. A third lost no water at all and grew seriously ill. Sickness occurred in other patients. Sometimes it was mild, but more frequently it involved headache, spots before the eyes, violent nausea, purging, and other discomforts. They were understandably frightened. They told Withering he could keep his medicine and they would keep their dropsy.

Withering did not know which way to turn. Digitalis worked, but there were obvious risks. His wife advised him not to take the chance of killing someone and ruining his medical career.

Decision was postponed when Withering was offered the opportunity to take over a fine Birmingham practice. He worked hard both in his practice and at the General Hospital. He made money and also a wealth of prominent friends.

One day his chief at the hospital, Dr. John Ash, inquired about the work he had done with digitalis. He asked to see Withering's notes. Withering confessed that, seeing twenty sick, poor patients an hour he had had no time for notes.

Ash then told him of a rather curious incident. A dropsy patient given up for dead had been cured with digitalis. The case might have gone unnoticed if the patient had not been a quite famous man, Dr. Cawley, head of one of the Oxford colleges.

Investigation revealed that Dr. Cawley had been given an immense dose of digitalis—twelve times as much as Withering had dared give any patient in the past. It was evidently time to look at digitalis again.

Withering was now a famous doctor. His patients would do anything he advised. There was ample opportunity to test digitalis on the many who had dropsy.

After several years of experimentation, Withering reached the conclusion that he was facing one of the trickiest dosage problems in medicine. There is no standard dosage for digitalis. What may be poison for one may be too weak a dose for another. Each patient has his particular need and his particular limit. This is equally true of the refined preparations in use today.

Withering was now carefully recording his cases—his successes and his failures. Most failures arose from the fact that, like Salmon half a century earlier, he believed that digitalis was a cure for tuberculosis as well as dropsy. But by 1779 he could point to five cures out of six. He permitted his findings, incomplete as they were, to be presented to the Edinburgh Medical Society. Scottish and English doctors asked themselves why they had refused to accept digitalis earlier.

In 1785 Withering felt it was time to make known his full conclusions. Many doctors who had heard of his work were using digitalis indiscriminately in the treatment of a number of diseases, including tuberculosis, for which he now knew it to be worthless. Those who were using it for dropsy were paying inadequate attention to the need for determining the proper dosage for each patient.

An Account of Foxglove appeared that year. In it Withering discussed 163 patients who took digitalis on his prescription. Of these, 101 had experienced relief. Analysis of the individual cases indicates that many of the remaining 62 were in fact suffering from problems that digitalis did not help.

Withering states in his *Account* that digitalis "has a power over the motion of the heart, to a degree yet unobserved in any other medicine, and that this power may be converted to salutary ends."[8] He did not, however, follow up this idea, and it seems unlikely that he thought of dropsy as being related to a malfunctioning of the heart.

Nevertheless, Withering made two important contributions. He recognized that the medical benefits of digitalis were limited to people suffering from dropsical retention of fluid. He found that the side effects of digitalis—the nausea and the vomiting—could be controlled by administering opium along with digitalis.

Withering was forty-four when he published his monumental work. He was already wasting away from tuberculosis which he had diagnosed in himself five years earlier. Despite increasing pain, he continued working to some extent until three years before his death in 1799.

A foxglove is carved on his monument at Old Church, Edgbaston.

DIGITALIS ACTS
ON THE HEART

Withering had plainly stated that digitalis was worthless in the treatment of tuberculosis. Nonetheless in the first quarter of the nineteenth century doctors continued to use it for this disease. An excuse that can be found for them is that they *wanted it to work*.

Less excusable was their persistence in ignoring Withering's directions about determining each patient's proper dosage. Instead, they pumped high overdoses into patients, often killing them. As a consequence, within thirty years of Withering's death digitalis had fallen back into disfavor.

But physicians who overdosed patients and regarded digitalis as a cure for tuberculosis were dying out by the close of the nineteenth century. Their places were being taken by young men with a thirst for knowledge. There was the Scotsman Arthur Robertson Cushny (1866-1926), who was professor of pharmacology successively at the universities of Michigan, London, and Edinburgh. Another Scotsman, James Mackenzie (1853-1925), started out as a simple family doctor only to become a distinguished English clinician. And there was Karel Frederik Wenckebach (1864-1940), resident physician at a Dutch old people's home (a good place to study heart disease) and professor of medicine at the University of Vienna from 1914 to 1929.

These men asked themselves: How does digitalis work? What does it do to the heart? Why do patients get dropsy? Why doesn't digitalis cure all dropsy patients?

Withering had observed that digitalis "has a power over the motion of the heart, to a degree yet unobserved in any other medicine." In 1799, John Ferriar said that "the power of reducing the pulse is the true characteristic" of digitalis. The same year, Thomas Beddoes found that digitalis "increases the organic action of the contractile fibers."[9] It is doubtful, however, whether any one of them recognized a direct connection between dropsy and weakness of the muscles of the upper heart. This was left to men like Cushny, Mackenzie, and Wenckebach.

In the years 1897 through 1925 Cushny did pioneer work on the effects of digitalis on the heart muscles. In 1902, William Einthoven (1860-1927) of the University of Leyden developed a string galvanometer that became the electrocardiograph. Cushny not only showed the value of the electrocardiogram in checking on the effects of digitalis but also modified the prevailing view of how digitalis operated.

In 1911, Cushny and Mackenzie, in experiments on dogs, demonstrated the wonderful efficacy of digitalis in atrial fibrillation, a disorder of the rhythm of the smaller chambers of the heart —the atria. Their work in elucidating the action of digitalis has been held "comparable to that of Withering in its discovery. [Their] experiment today is the centerpiece of our knowledge of the action of digitalis. . . ."[10]

Atrial fibrillation has the effect of changing the regular, pumping action of the heart into a faint, uneven squirting. This irregular action is unable to push blood fast enough through the arteries and veins. Blood accumulates in the major vessels and a watery fluid swells arms, legs, chest, and belly. This condition used to be called dropsy. It is now known as edema.

A fibrillation is actually a tremor that upsets the heart rhythm. Cushny and Mackenzie found that digitalis overcame the effect of the tremor and permitted the heart to resume its powerful pumping action. The revitalized circulation picks up fluid from the swollen tissue and carries it to the kidneys, whence it is flushed out of the body.

In short, digitalis acts on the heart as a stimulant. It does not *dry* surplus fluid out of the body as had long been supposed. Its effect on accumulated fluid is indirect. Dr. Salerne of Orleans, who observed that his overdosed turkeys had been squeezed out like a sponge, attributed this to the *direct* action of foxglove leaves. Others followed in this belief.

The fact that digitalis operates on the heart explains why it did not cure all cases of dropsy. While a majority of edemas or dropsies result from atrial fibrillation or congestive heart failure, there are other causes. These include obstruction of the lymph vessels, disturbances in kidney functioning, and a reduction in plasma proteins. Digitalis does nothing to relieve the patient's suffering when the heart is not involved.

In 1910 Mackenzie had brought the fight for the acceptance of digitalis to Harley Street, the center of arch-conservatism. He lost. His fellow specialists continued to let their patients die rather than adopt a "new-fangled remedy" that had in fact been recommended to "scatter the dropsy" back in the sixteenth century. Mackenzie became famous, but for what he regarded as his lesser achievements. He, Cushny, and Wenckebach retired and died. But they had students who took up and finally won their battle.

One problem remained. Digitalis had had a long history of toxicity. Therefore, it was customary to stop administering the drug just as soon as symptoms of cardiac insufficiency lessened. A course of digitalis treatment would run for a week or two at most. In a majority of cases, the symptoms would return in a matter of weeks or months. Then emergency treatment with digitalis would be repeated.

At length, under the leadership of such men as Joseph H. Pratt and Henry Jackson, both of Harvard Medical School, the practice of short-term administration of digitalis was abandoned in favor of continued administration, if necessary for many years.

It was said at the beginning of this discussion that dropsy occurs so infrequently today that most of us have never seen a case of it. Why, then, is there a continuing need for digitalis?

The best explanation is that the field has been reversed. For thousands of years dropsy was a killer and no one knew that it had any connection with the functioning of the heart. Withering recognized that there was a connection two centuries ago, but he was still treating dropsy. Today we know that dropsy or edema is an outcome of heart irregularity. It might be said that digitalis is now more often used to prevent dropsy than to cure it.

The patient is digitalized at the first sign of cardiac insufficiency and in most cases edema does not follow. In short, digitalis was originally considered a dropsy drug and is now recognized as a heart drug.

A PURIFIED PRODUCT
BUT STILL DIGITALIS

In 1869, C. A. Nativelle of France discovered the active principle in digitalis. It was a sugar that he named *digitalin*. A few years later it was "rediscovered" by Oswald Schmiedeberg of Germany, who called it *digitoxin*. Today we have in addition *lanoxin* (or *digoxin*), *gitalin, ouabain,* and several other drugs less commonly in use.

All these preparations are glycosides of digitalis or related plants. A glycoside is any substance obtained from plants which, when treated hydrolytically, produces a sugar and other products.

While some doctors still prefer standardized preparations of digitalis, such as the powdered leaf or a diluted alcohol solution, the pure drug has today been largely replaced by the purified glycosides, which can be injected or given orally in more accurately determined doses. The glycosides are also less apt to cause intestinal upset.

In 1785, Withering wrote in *An Account of the Foxglove:*

"TIME will fix the real value upon this discovery, and determine whether I have imposed upon myself and others, or contributed to the benefit of science and mankind."[11]

Time has not only more than justified Withering's digitalis; it has revealed what is not true of many folk medicines that have been adopted as modern drugs. It would seem that it is not possible to produce chemically a synthetic that will do the job of digitalis. The glycosides, while refined, are still derived from the leaves of the foxglove.

Without the faith and work of Withering and those who followed him, we might today stand helpless in the face of many heart problems.

Seven

The
Accidental Miracle
⌐ Penicillin

MOLDY
BREAD

The folk medicines considered up to this point have all come from plants or the barks of trees. But there is in addition a form of plant life that is so primitive that it can have no independent existence. Members of this plant family are parasites that rely on other organisms, living or dead, for their food. Yet these far from helpless fungi, as they are called, are the source of one of the most effective remedies known to modern medical science. At the same time, some of them are poisonous and cause sickness or death. This of course is true of other plants that have medicinal value.

The fungi operate to break down and transform organic and inorganic matter. The effects of their activity can be either beneficial or destructive. On the positive side, fungi are responsible for the development of lifesaving drugs and are harnessed for the commercial production of mushrooms and Roquefort and Camembert cheese. The negative side involves the spoilage of food, the rotting of fabric, and undesirable physical conditions such as athlete's foot.

Perhaps the fungi we are most familiar with are those that appear as mildew or in the form of molds on various foods. We have all seen at one time or another the blue-green mold that develops on bread. Mushrooms and toadstools are also fungi, but of a different order.

The placing of moldy bread on cuts was a country remedy long before anyone had heard of penicillin. For just how long is an

145

interesting question. The practice may even date back to 2900 B.C. and to the first physician whose name has come down in history, the Egyptian Imhotep. In any event, moldy wheaten bread was used by the ancient Egyptians in the treatment of cases involving skin eruptions and was possibly one of the most active therapeutic substances known in the ancient world. Wheaten flour and wheaten bread showed up as the "most effective ingredient" in a number of Egyptian remedies, including problems connected with the bladder and other urinary organs.

It is possible, of course, that the Egyptians thought that the curative factor was the wheat flour. Mold forms so rapidly on bread, meat, and other foods in climates like Egypt's that it would be easy to imagine that the parasite was an integral part of the parent. But we now recognize that the effective agent was the antibacterial activity of *Penicillium,* the family of which bread mold is a member.

The Egyptians were not alone among early peoples to use molds in medical treatment. The Chinese treated boils, carbuncles, and infected wounds with molds and soy-flour poultices. In India, mold was a remedy for dysentery, a condition involving bacterial infection. American Indians used molds for wounds suffered in battle, and there is evidence of a similar use by the Mayans of Central America. Hippocrates recommended toasted molds for the treatment of certain female disorders. In the Middle Ages, the wound of a lord returning from a foray or hunting trip was covered by his lady with a poultice of moldy bread and hot yeast (a form of fungus) or sprinkled with powdered mushrooms. In the twelfth century, Hildegard of Bingen, the abbess who condemned colchicum, wrote: "The sponges and fungi that grow on dead and living trees can in many instances be eaten and they are good as medicine."[1]

Then for some centuries there was little mention of fungi in medical literature. Between the mid-seventeenth century and the late nineteenth century there was practically none at all.

THE CRITICAL
BACKGROUND

From the sixteenth century B.C. and possibly earlier, molds were used in the treatment of external and internal infection *because they worked*. The Hindu, Chinese, and Egyptian physicians had found that bread poultices were effective. It didn't matter whether the actual agent was the flour, the adherent mold, a combination of the two, or some totally unrecognized factor. Their approach was empirical. That is, it was based on experience and observation alone and did not rely on theory or an established system. Even those who recognized mold as the active principle had no idea why it worked or what it worked on or against.

A remedy for which no more substantial justification could be offered was bound to be weak in staying power. This at least partly explains why this ancient practice fell from grace as the world emerged from the Middle Ages, even though poultices of moldy bread undoubtedly continued in use among those who saw no doctors.

Empiric remedies were all very well, but the establishment of specific remedies called for predetermination of the causes of specific infections. In the fifth century B.C. Hippocrates had proclaimed his theory of the imbalance of the four humors as the cause of illness and miasmas (bad air) as a spreader of infection, especially in the case of epidemics. These principles dominated medical thought and practice at least up to the sixteenth century A.D. Disease germs played no part in the Hippocratic schema. Until the concept of disease germs was accepted, a large number of diseases remained untreatable.

An important contribution was made by the Italian physician

(and poet) Girolamo Fracastoro. When Columbus returned from the West Indies in 1493, his crew was believed to have brought back a previously unknown disease, now called syphilis. There is evidence today to suggest that the crew was wrongly blamed, but whatever its origin the "great pox," as it was then called, had spread throughout Europe twenty-five years later. It was common among patients of Fracastoro. He observed that it invariably passed from one individual to another *by contact*—not through the air as Hippocrates and his followers would have it.

This prompted Fracastoro to turn his attention to other diseases. He found that either contagion or bodily contact (or both) was involved in the passing on of such epidemic diseases as cholera, plague, and smallpox. Hippocrates's bad-air theory, he said, had been misleading and incomplete. Before there could be an epidemic, there had to be a source, a "prepared field." The disease seed was "raised" in this prepared field which was, of course, the individual who would pass on the disease. After it was raised, the infectious matter could be passed on by contact. Fracastoro thus established the concept of the disease seed. He set up a signpost that would help guide others to the recognition of bacteria as a prime cause of infection.

But the science of bacteriology could never have developed out of what physicians might see with their naked eye, however brilliant the conclusions they drew. It was necessary to see the seed, and the seed—the bacterium—was the most minute of living particles.

It is hard to say just who invented the microscope. Pliny the Elder had written in A.D. 77 of "burning glasses" that might be "spherical or lens-shaped." Somewhat earlier, Seneca had announced that letters, however minute and obscure, are seen larger and clearer through a glass bulb filled with water. The tenth-century Arabian physicist Ibn-al-Haytham or Alhazen described the magnifying power of a lens in his *Optics*. In the thirteenth century, Roger Bacon spoke of a reading lens "useful to old men and those having feeble sight. For they can see a letter or anything small in sufficient size." A tomb in the Church of Santa Maria Maggiore in Florence is inscribed, "Here lies Salvino Darmato degli Armati of Florence, inventor of spectacles. God pardon his sins. A.D. 1317." Undoubtedly all of these "inventions" contributed to the development of the microscope.[2] But primary credit is often given to Johannes Jansen and his son Zacharias of Middelburg, Holland. The Jansens were spectacle makers. About 1590, they discovered that two convex lenses placed at a proper distance from each other produced high magnification. Word of this discovery spread to Italy where, in 1624, Galileo constructed a microscope (in addition to his better-known telescope). Several years elapsed before the microscope was adopted in medical studies.

Athanasius Kircher (1598-1680) was born in the small town of Geisa in what is now East Germany. He became a Jesuit and a professor at the universities of Würzburg and Rome. During an outbreak of plague in Europe, he removed a drop of fluid from a draining plague sore. He examined it under the best microscope then available. He described "minute worms which were capable of propagation . . . so thin, so small, so tiny, that it passes our comprehension unless we observe them through the best available microscope."[3] In a report published in Leipzig in 1659 he named these creatures *contagium animatum*—"living contagion." He maintained that they were responsible for all communicable diseases in man. Unfortunately nobody paid attention and 235 years passed before Yersin and Kitasato isolated the plague bacillus, which Kircher had apparently observed.

Fortunately more attention was paid the microscopical observations of Anton van Leeuwenhoek (1632-1723). This Dutch merchant had a hobby of grinding lenses and constructing microscopes. At one time he was said to possess 237 microscopes that he had made. For the last fifty years of his life he conscientiously reported his findings to the Royal Society of London.

In one of his early reports he described incredibly small animals observed in lake water that had been left standing a few days to form a skin on its surface. "They stop and collect at one point, then they suddenly turn in a circle as fast as a spinning top, and the circle in which they move is no larger than a grain of sand."[4]

Two years later he set out to determine why pepper was so "sharp," as he put it. He crushed a peppercorn in water. After it had stood awhile, his microscope revealed a very large number of "little animals" so small that "a coarse grain of sand could hold a million of them, and there must have been at least 2,700,-000 living in a drop of pepper water."[5]

In 1683 he examined tartar from his own and other people's teeth and saw what would later be classified as cocci, bacilli, filamentous forms, and spirochetes. He drew pictures of them as he saw them: "short, straight rods, balls, curved rods and spiral ones that look like corkscrews."[6]

The "disease seed" about which Fracastoro had speculated had at last been seen. It was named *bacterium* from the Greek *bakterion* meaning a stick, rod, or little rod; the name seems to have first been used by C. G. Ehrenburg (1795-1876) in a book published in 1838.

Gustav Jakob Henle (1809-1885), a German histologist, published a book called *The Formation of Pus and Mucus* in 1838. He reported in it that microscopic examination had revealed very small living creatures in diseased tissue that were not present in healthy tissue. He proposed the hypothesis that these creatures were the cause of numerous diseases and laid down the basic principles by which bacteria could be clearly implicated in specific diseases.

In 1870, the German botanist Ferdinand Cohn (1828-1898) showed that bacteria belong in the plant kingdom and laid the foundations for the present system of classifying bacteria. Then, in 1876, the German bacteriologist Robert Koch (1843-1910) and Louis Pasteur (1822-1895), France's greatest scientist, demonstrated that the disease anthrax was invariably associated with a specific form of bacilli. This was the first clear proof that a disease was caused by a species of bacteria. At the same time Koch developed Henle's principles for implicating specific bacteria in specific diseases. Guided by these elaborated principles, since known as "Koch's postulates," Pasteur, Koch, and their associates isolated the pathogenic organisms in a series of diseases. Perhaps most dramatic of all was Koch's isolation of the dreaded tubercle bacillus. These remarkable successes seemed to promise the opening of a new era in medicine. And so they did, from the standpoint of *preventive* medicine. If the pathogenic bacteria could be prevented from reaching the potential host, these bacterial diseases could be prevented. However, there remained the question of what could be done once bacteria had invaded a patient.

JOSEPH LISTER AND THE DEVELOPMENT OF ANTISEPSIS

Even before these issues had become clearly defined, the British surgeon Joseph Lister (1827-1912) had attempted to prevent pathogenic organisms from invading his patients and to destroy organisms which already had invaded. The departure point for his ideas was Pasteur's work on fermentation in the 1850s and 1860s. Following up earlier suggestions that alcoholic fermentation was associated with the activity of living yeast cells, Pasteur demonstrated that air-borne living organisms could produce a series of different fermentations. Since some scientists had long believed that fermentation, putrefaction, and infection were fundamentally similar processes, Lister reasoned that infection, like fermentation, might be caused by air-borne living organisms. If these organisms could be kept away from patients' wounds—or destroyed once they reached them—perhaps the lethal danger of infection could be eliminated.

Lister established a routine based on these ideas. He sought a nonpoisonous and antiseptic substance that would keep air-borne organisms away from the wound, destroy those that might reach the site of the wound, and at the same time do no harm to the patient. First, the wound and the area around it were cleansed with carbolic acid, a corrosive substance lethal to microorganisms—that is, an *anti-septic* substance. Then the wound was covered with oiled silk to prevent the bandage from sticking to it. Finally, eight layers of gauze soaked in carbolic acid were topped by a waterproof covering designed to slow evaporation and keep the gauze moist. In this way he effectively sealed off the wound from outside influences. Results over a nine-month period beginning in 1865 were encouraging, despite the facts that Lister did not know precisely what he was protecting the wound from and that carbolic acid was often irritating and harmful to the human tissues to which it was applied.

More dramatically successful was Lister's later practice of spraying the operating room with carbolic acid during surgery. This largely prevented the extremely common postoperative infection which was the bane of surgeons of that time. It was particularly for this development in antiseptic surgery that Lister won his fame.

STEPS TOWARD
PENICILLIN, 1871-1900

In 1871, Lister stumbled on a phenomenon, which, if he could have interpreted it, might have brought him even greater fame. In an attempt to trap air-borne bacteria, he had set up six containers, each filled with one-half ounce of nutrient broth. He had covered two of the containers immediately; two he left uncovered for a couple of days; the remaining two he never covered. After four days he found to his disappointment that five of the containers were free of growth. The sixth had grown a fine lawn on its surface—a mold. Lister decided to find out what would happen if he introduced bacteria to this mold.

He divided the growth of fine lawn between two dishes, with by far the greater amount in one of them. He added a number of disease bacteria to each. "Both exhibited bacteria in abundance," he reported, "but there was a marked difference between them as regards their activity," The bacteria in the dish containing the small amount of lawn "exhibited the most amazing energy." Those in the other dish "were comparatively languid, multitudes were entirely motionless."[7] From this evidence, the superficial conclusion to be drawn was simply that the bacteria were too much for the mold in the one case and the mold was too much for the bacteria in the other. But surely it was significant that the mold had stopped the bacteria, even if only in one case? Unaccountably, Lister seems to have dropped the investigation at this point.

It is hard to say why Lister failed to realize that he was on the track of an antibacterial that would prove even more important than carbolic acid. Perhaps he was put off by the fact that the mold seemed only to stupefy rather than to kill the bacteria. Perhaps his mind was so fixed on his antiseptic that he found it hard to think in terms of other approaches to bacteria control. The fact remains that he had observed what Alexander Fleming would "discover" and name "penicillin" fifty-seven years later.

Lister was not alone in observing the action of *Penicillium* on certain bacteria. In 1876 the British physicist John Tyndall (1820-1893) was attempting to explode the theory of the spontaneous generation of living substances. In one experiment he confined bacteria and *Penicillium glaucum* in the same test tube. A thick, tough layer of mold sealed off the mouth of the test tube. The bacteria lost their power to reproduce and fell dead or dormant at the bottom of the tube. After describing this action of *Penicillium* mold, Tyndall concluded that the blocking of the mouth of the tube by the mold had shut off "the oxygen necessary to Bacterial life."[8] Though not unreasonable, his conclusion left unexplored the possibility that the mold itself was antibacterial.

In 1877, Pasteur was studying the rate of growth of different strains of bacteria. Ordinarily, he grew each strain in a separate dish. However, one day he found himself with a limited supply of nutrient broth. Not wishing to interrupt his program, he placed three different types of bacteria in the same dish. He believed that each would have sufficient space to grow in and expected that they would pay no attention to each other. To his surprise, none of them did well. This led Pasteur to the conclusion that "life hinders life,"[9] an observation that was greatly to influence the later development of antibacterials.

At the end of the century, Ernest Duchesne, a young man up for his medical degree at the Army Academy at Lyon, France, was inspired by Pasteur to study bacteria.

Duchesne made three fundamental observations.

First, the air was full of fungi. If a single spore fell on a piece of bread, stale fruit, cheese, or jam, the food was soon covered with a thick growth of mold.

Second, there were no fungi in the cultures in which he grew his bacteria.

Third, mold viewed under a microscope revealed no trace of bacteria.

Duchesne decided that in the one situation the bacteria were the stronger and the fungi had to yield, while in the other the bacteria retreated in the face of stronger fungi. Or, as Pasteur had stated it, "Life hinders life."

Duchesne cultivated *Penicillium glaucum,* a fungus that creates particularly healthy colonies on a piece of moist bread. First, it formed a wide mat. Then a layer of bluish-green-gray spore heads developed on top of it.

Duchesne introduced to this fungus some bacteria ordinarily found in the intestines. The bacteria were dead within a matter of hours.

Next he vaccinated some white mice with the intestinal bacteria and others with typhoid bacteria. Half the mice were then injected with nutrient broth on which fungus had been grown.

The following day, all mice that had received fungus broth were alive and well; neither bacteria had harmed them in any way. The rest of the mice were dead. Duchesne concluded that fungi could master bacteria even within the body.

The twenty-one-year-old Frenchman wrote a thesis reporting his discoveries. It was ignored. He became an army doctor and forgot his scientific ambitions.

The situation was ironic in more ways than one. This man who had great potential as a researcher wound up examining blistered feet. He had approached a problem scientifically and his solution had been ignored. The ultimate discoverer of penicillin would do so "by chance"—and not for another thirty years.

THE ACTUAL
DISCOVERY

The Scotsman Alexander Fleming (1881-1955) was in his early thirties at the outbreak of World War I. The next four years found him attempting to heal infected war wounds. This experience aroused in him an interest in staphylococcic infection that would remain with him throughout his professional career.

He had observed that the white corpuscles in the blood did a heroic job battling and even overcoming infection. He concluded that these white corpuscles or leucocytes must possess an active substance that set in motion and stimulated the defense mechanism of the body. Actually, he was laying the foundation both for the modern concept of antibodies that spring to the defense at any invasion of the body and for the concept of immune reaction—rejection—as it has become familiar in transplant procedures.

The importance of Fleming's deduction cannot be overestimated. Even today, the miracle drugs—penicillin, the sulfas, and the mycetins—only operate to break the first line of bacterial offense. Thereafter, the leucocytes take over and finish the job.

Fleming decided to search for the active substance in leucocytes. In 1922, four years after the war had ended, his continuing research was rewarded by the discovery of an enzyme in the white blood cells that was capable of destroying bacteria. He named this enzyme *lysozyme*.

This discovery encouraged him to look further into the activities of bacteria. In 1928 he was working in a modest laboratory at St. Mary's Hospital, London, on staphylococci—the germs that cause pimples, boils, carbuncles, and sometimes serious blood infections.

On a gloomy September afternoon his assistant had prepared a series of petri dishes containing staphylococci cultures for incubation at body temperature. Two days later, Fleming found that the staphylococci had spread like a smooth lawn over the nutrient surface of all the dishes but one. In this, there were dull-looking islands of staphylococci while the rest of the surface was dotted with a greenish-gray fungus. His assistant was under standing orders to cover all dishes as soon as they were prepared. Obviously this single dish had been left uncovered long enough for a spore to alight out of the smoky murk that formed at nearby Paddington railroad station.

Since the staphylococci growth was full on all the other dishes, Fleming could conclude that the intruder was in some way destroying the bacteria. But how? Evidently the fungus was not making a direct attack. There were islands of cocci and islands of fungi separated by clear nutrient. Fleming supposed that the fungus was introducing some lethal substance into the nutrient.

Fleming decided to name this substance *penicillin*. He took the name directly from the genus name for such fungi—*Penicillium,* which derives from the Latin word *penicillus* meaning a brush; the minute spore-bearing stems of fungi have brushlike projections at the tips.

A specialist in fungi wrongly identified Fleming's fungus as *Penicillium rubrum*. It was in fact *Penicillium notatum*. But the mycologist may be forgiven his error. Few men of his science can positively identify one out of the thousands of different species of *Penicillium* that exist.

Fleming reported his discovery as an odd laboratory experience. It would later be recognized as a historic achievement, but for a dozen years it was to lie buried in what has been described as "the graveyard of small print in a laboratory journal."[10]

Fleming continued his experiments with penicillin for ten years. He soon satisfied himself that penicillin was effective against staphylococci, pneumococci, gonococci, streptococci, and a number of other disease bacteria. At the same time he determined that penicillin did not attack all bacteria but left a part of the field open to the sulfa drugs and the mycetins. He concluded in an article published in June 1929 that "penicillin may be an antiseptic effective upon application on, or injection into, the areas infected by microbes sensitive to its action."[11]

Almroth Edward Wright (1861-1947), who in the 1890s pioneered antityphoid vaccination, had been Fleming's teacher. He had pounded into his students that every bacteriological discovery must be judged by its effects on the human body.

Fleming knew the course he should follow. But he was a bacteriologist, not a practicing physician. In his view, experiments on humans were not for the bacteriologist. Besides, he knew from his medical training that only pure penicillin should be given to the patient. The best that he and his assistant could produce was a decanted fungal culture that, in addition to penicillin, included residual broth and God knew what else.

Fleming had previously experimented with a number of anti-bacterials. All of them had destroyed the life-insuring leucocytes as well as bacteria. Now, when Fleming tried out his penicillin broth on rabbits with infected wounds, it not only had a healing effect but, more importantly, the leucocytes, the defense mechanisms of the body were not affected by the treatment. Penicillin was definitely not "poisonous." Yet Fleming still hesitated to try it on humans. That, he decided, must be left to others. He withdrew into his bacteriological shell and lost himself in a study of the influenza bacillus.

An occasional colleague experimented with penicillin in the sterilization of wounds. The results were often disappointing. One doctor summed up his experience in these words: "The penicillium moulds are pleasant enough and we are content to use them to bring our Camembert and Roquefort cheeses into a pleasant condition of ripeness, and in that respect I would not like to miss them. But beyond that, and especially with a view to therapy in medicine, these moulds are completely useless."[12]

FURTHER RESEARCH
AT OXFORD

Howard Walter Florey (1898-1968) was born in Adelaide, Australia. At Cambridge University in England he experimented with all sorts of substances that he thought might kill bacteria, becoming acquainted with Fleming's lysozyme. By 1939 he was a professor at the Sir William Dunn School of Pathology at Oxford. Among his co-workers were his wife, Ethel, also a doctor; a young American, Leslie Falk; Norman Heatley, an English microbiologist; and Ernst Boris Chain, a thirty-three-year-old refugee from Hitler's Germany (who with Fleming and Florey was to be awarded the Nobel Prize in medicine and physiology in 1945 for their work on penicillin).

This Oxford group was trying to produce pure lysozyme in the laboratory. They finally succeeded, producing a synthetic that killed bacteria just as Fleming's lysozyme had done. Then they went in search of other products harmless to man but deadly to bacteria.

Their search led them to Fleming's 1929 article in which he had reported his success and disappointments with penicillin. Chain studied the report and then ordered spores of *Penicillium notatum* from Fleming's London laboratory. He started growing the fungus and, with his co-workers, embarked on a series of experiments. The bacteriologists looked for the best conditions under which the fungus would grow. They attempted to determine the chemical structure of penicillin. "To make any start here," Florey said, "it will be necessary to produce an entirely pure product."[13] To which Heatley added: "What we need is a unit measure by which we will know the amount of penicillin, in the same way we now know the temperature of the room by looking at the thermometer, or the distance between two points by using a yardstick."[14] By 1941 the group had established its measure and, after successful experimentation with animals, had accumulated enough of a yellow-brown powder that was pure penicillin to test on man.

The person selected was a London bobby who was dying from staphylococcic and streptococcic infections. Sulfa drugs had done nothing for him.

On February 12, 1941, when the policeman had been hospitalized for five months, Florey decided to inject penicillin into his bloodstream. His condition improved within twenty-four hours. By February 17, there was every reason to expect he would recover. Then the supply of penicillin ran out. The process of growing fungi and extracting penicillin was slow and the quantity produced meager. The patient died a month later.

PRODUCTION
IN AMERICA

World War II was in its second year. Penicillin was in great demand for the treatment of the wounded and there was no supply of it anywhere. In the summer of 1941 Florey and Heatley came to America in the hope of getting penicillin produced in quantity.

The *Penicillium notatum* that the British scientists brought with them was a slow, plodding mold that produced only two units of penicillin for each cubic centimeter of the nutrient on which it grew. Investigators at the Department of Agriculture Laboratory in Peoria, Illinois, found a mold strain of *Penicillium chrysogenum* that produced 100 units per cubic centimeter. The strain came from rotten cantaloupes.

It was next found that corn-steep liquor, a waste substance from the manufacture of cornstarch, stimulated the mold to a still greater yield. (Corn-steep liquor is still used by the carload in the manufacture of penicillin.)

The British growing method had involved a jellied medium. This was abandoned in favor of a liquid medium composed of water, proteins, salts, and sugars. Whiskey flasks, milk bottles, and all sorts of glass containers were commandeered wherever they could be found. A production and speed record was established by penicillin raised in flasks at a small mushroom plant in West Chester, Pennsylvania. By August 1943, thanks to the unnamed thousands of Americans who contributed in a variety of ways, enough penicillin was being produced to save millions of lives. First call was for our war casualties and those of our allies. Penicillin was then a crude drug varying in color from dark brown to canary yellow to pale yellow. The white crystalline penicillin that we have come to know as the "white magic" came later, after long hours of hard work on the part of American chemists.

Poppies, foxglove, meadow saffron, the coca bush, willow and cinchona trees, and fungi are not the only plants that grow in the medical garden. However, some of the modern drugs most important in the preservation of health are the ones derived from these seven. What they have in common, apart from being plant life, is that they started out long ago as folk remedies.

Today, doctors prescribe multicolored capsules or tablets that look as if they had been developed yesterday. Patients do not stop to think of the years of trial and error that lie behind these drugs. Yet, like many things in everyday life, they have a history that puts modern technology in perspective and lessens the mystery of a highly mechanized existence.

Reference Notes
Selected Bibliography
Index

Reference Notes

One: "The Plant of Good and Evil"

1   J. M. Scott, *The White Poppy* (New York: Funk & Wagnalls, 1969), p. 6.
2   *Ibid.*, p. 7.
3   Soheil M. Afnan, *Avicenna, His Life and Works* (London: George Allen and Unwin Ltd., 1958), p. 75.
4   Henry E. Sigerist, *Paracelsus After Four Hundred Years,* in Félix Martí-Ibáñez (ed.), *Henry E. Sigerist on the History of Medicine* (New York: MD Publications, 1960), p. 167.
5   *Ibid.*, p. 172.
6   Charles H. LaWall, *Four Thousand Years of Pharmacy* (Philadelphia and London: Lippincott, 1927), p. 262.
7   *Ibid.*, p. 281.
8   *Ibid.*
9   Milton Silverman, *Magic in a Bottle* (2nd ed. New York: Macmillan, 1948), p. 2.
10 *Ibid.*, p. 10.
11 *Ibid.*
12 *Ibid.*, p. 11.
13 *Ibid.*, p. 15.
14 *Ibid.*
15 James D. Watson, *The Double Helix* (New York: Atheneum, 1968), p. 4.
16 Arthur Dickson Wright, "The History of Opium," *Medical and Biological Illustration,* XVIII (January 1968), p. 68.
17 "3-nation war on boom in dope," *Chicago Daily News,* May 2-3, 1970, p. 3.

18   "Kids and Heroin: The Adolescent," *Time,* March 16, 1970, p. 16.
19   Scott, *op. cit.,* p. 127.
20   *Ibid.,* p. 131.
21   *Ibid.,* p. 125.
22   *Ibid.,* p. 1.

Two: The Divine Plant of the Incas

1   Silverman, *Magic in a Bottle,* p. 91.
2   *Ibid.*
3   H. Blejer-Prieto, "Coca Leaf and Cocaine Addiction—Some Historical Notes," *Canadian Medical Association Journal,* XCIII (September 25, 1965), p. 701.
4   Hortense Koller Becker, "Carl Koller and Cocaine," *The Psychoanalytic Quarterly,* XXXII (1963), p. 321.
5   Silverman, *op. cit.,* p. 97.
6   Blejer-Prieto, *op. cit.,* p. 703.
7   Francis Darwin, *Eugenics Review* (1914), cited by William Osler in *Proceedings of the Royal Society of Medicine,* XI (1918), p. 66.
8   Silverman, *op. cit.,* p. 103.
9   *Ibid.,* p. 104.
10   *Ibid.,* pp. 105-106.
11   Blejer-Prieto, *loc. cit.*
12   Silverman, *op. cit.,* p. 110.
13   David F. Musto, "A Study in Cocaine—Sherlock Holmes and Sigmund Freud," *Journal of the American Medical Association,* CCIV (April 1, 1968), p. 31.
14   *Ibid.,* p. 28.
15   Silverman, *op. cit.,* pp. 110-111.
16   "How to teach a 5-year-old about drugs so he'll listen," *Chicago Daily News,* October 17-18, 1970, p. 5.

Three: The Powder of the Countess

1 Silverman, *Magic in a Bottle,* p. 27; M. L. Duran-Reynals, *The Fever Bark Tree* (New York: Doubleday, 1946), p. 24.
2 Duran-Reynals, *op. cit.,* p. 4.
3 *Ibid.,* p. 9.
4 *Ibid.,* p. 13.
5 *Ibid.*
6 *Ibid.,* pp. 17-18.
7 *Ibid.,* p. 72.
8 Silverman, *op. cit.,* p. 30.
9 Ralph H. Major, *A History of Medicine* (2 vols. Springfield, Ill.: Thomas, 1954), I, 550.
10 Duran-Reynals, *op. cit.,* p. 90.
11 Edith Grey Wheelwright, *The Physick Garden* (London: Jonathan Cape, 1934), p. 153.
12 Duran-Reynals, *op. cit.,* p. 181.
13 Thomas Findley, "Sappington's Anti-Fever Pills and the Westward Migration," *Transactions, American Clinical and Climatological Association,* LXXIX (1967), p. 36.
14 *Ibid.*
15 H. A. Martin, "Notes on Quinine," *Pharmaceutical Journal,* X (1900), p. 337.

Four: The Remedy in Every Medicine Cabinet

1 Silverman, *Magic in a Bottle,* p. 149.
2 *Ibid.,* p. 152.
3 *Ibid.*
4 *Ibid.,* p. 154.
5 *Ibid.,* p. 155.

Five: Calming a Swollen Toe

1 W. S. C. Copeman, *A Short History of Gout and the Rheumatic Diseases* (Berkeley: University of California Press, 1964), pp. 41-42.

2 Thomas Sydenham, "A Treatise of the Gout," *Medical Classics,* IV (1939), p. 363.

3 Copeman, *op. cit.,* p. 39.

4 Major, *A History of Medicine,* I, 283.

5 Copeman, *op. cit.,* p. 41.

6 *Ibid.,* p. 43.

7 *Ibid.,* p. 44.

8 *Ibid.,* p. 45.

9 Maurice A. Schnitker, "A History of the Treatment of Gout," *Bulletin of the History of Medicine,* IV (1936), p. 105.

10 Carl Van Doren, *Benjamin Franklin* (New York: Viking, 1938), p. 361.

11 *Ibid.,* p. 493.

12 *Ibid.,* p. 770.

13 William Pepper, *The Medical Side of Benjamin Franklin* (Philadelphia: Campbell, 1911), p. 90.

14 James Moore, "A Letter to Dr. Jones on the Composition of Eau Médicinale," *New England Journal of Medicine and Surgery,* I (1812), p. 97.

Six: A Cure for Dropsy

1 J. Worth Estes and Paul Dudley White, "William Withering and the Purple Foxglove" *Scientific American,* CCXII (1965), p. 111.

2 *Ibid.,* p. 112.

3 Silverman, *Magic in a Bottle,* p. 61.

4 Major, *A History of Medicine,* I, 492.

5 Fielding H. Garrison, *An Introduction to the History of Medicine* (4th ed. Philadelphia and London: Saunders, 1929), p. 231.
6 Silverman, *op. cit.,* p. 64.
7 Estes and White, *loc. cit.*
8 William Withering, *An Account of the Foxglove, and Some of Its Medical Uses, with Practical Remarks on Dropsy, and Other Diseases* (Birmingham: Robinson, 1785), p. 192.
9 Estes and White, *op. cit.,* p. 115.
10 John C. Krantz, Jr., C. Jelleff Carr, *The Pharmacological Principles of Medical Practice* (7th ed. Baltimore: Williams and Wilkins, 1969), p. 119.
11 Withering, *op. cit.,* p. x.

Seven: The Accidental Miracle

1 Helmuth M. Böttcher, *Miracle Drugs* (London: Heinemann, 1963), p. 108.
2 Major, *A History of Medicine,* I, 507-8.
3 Böttcher, *op. cit.,* p. 114.
4 *Ibid.,* p. 115.
5 *Ibid.,* p. 116.
6 *Ibid.*
7 *Ibid.,* p. 131.
8 Henry Welch and Félix Martí-Ibáñez, *The Antibiotic Saga* (New York: Medical Encyclopedia, 1960), p. 19.
9 Böttcher, *op. cit.,* p. 136.
10 Welch and Martí-Ibáñez, *op. cit.,* pp. 14-15.
11 *Ibid.,* p. 16.
12 Böttcher, *op. cit.,* p. 157.
13 *Ibid.,* p. 161.
14 *Ibid.,* p. 162.

Selected Bibliography

Becker, Hortense Koller. "Carl Koller and Cocaine," *The Psycho-analytic Quarterly,* XXXII (1963), pp. 309-373.

Blejer-Prieto, H. "Coca Leaf and Cocaine Addiction—Some Historical Notes," *Canadian Medical Association Journal,* XCIII (September 25, 1965), pp. 700-703.

Böttcher, Helmuth M. *Miracle Drugs.* London: Heinemann, 1963.

Copeman, W. S. C. *A Short History of the Gout and Rheumatic Diseases.* Berkeley: University of California Press, 1964.

Duran-Reynals, M. L. *The Fever Bark Tree.* New York: Doubleday, 1946.

Estes, T. Worth, and White, Paul Dudley. "William Withering and the Purple Foxglove," *Scientific American,* CCXII (1965), 110-116, 119.

Findley, Thomas. "Sappington's Anti-Fever Pills and the Westward Migration," *Transactions, American Clinical and Climatological Association,* LXXIX (1967), 34-44.

Fitzgerald, William J. "Evolution of the Use of Quinine in Treatment of Malaria," *New York State Journal of Medicine,* LXVIII (1968), 800-802.

LaWall, Charles H. *Four Thousand Years of Pharmacy.* Philadelphia and London: Lippincott, 1927.

Major, Ralph H. *A History of Medicine,* 2 vols. Springfield, Ill.: Thomas, 1954.

Musto, David F. "A Study of Cocaine—Sherlock Holmes and Sigmund Freud," *Journal of the American Medical Association,* CCIV (April 1, 1968), 27-32.

Scott, J. M. *The White Poppy.* New York: Funk & Wagnalls, 1969.

171

Silverman, Milton. *Magic in a Bottle*. 2nd ed. New York: Macmillan, 1948.

Van Doren, Carl. *Benjamin Franklin*. New York: Viking, 1938.

Wallace, Stanley L. "Benjamin Franklin and the Introduction of Colchicum into the United States," *Bulletin of the History of Medicine*, XLII (July-August 1968), 312-320.

Welch, Henry, and Martí-Ibáñez, Félix. *The Antibiotic Saga*. New York: Medical Encyclopedia, 1960.

Wright, Arthur Dickson. "The History of Opium," *Medical and Biological Illustration*. XVIII (January 1968), 62-70.

Index

About the Authors

Geoffrey Marks was born in Australia and received his B.A. (1928) and M.A. (1940) from Trinity College, Oxford. Now a United States citizen, he is Associate Editor of *Physician's Management* and the author of *The Medieval Plague* and *The Amazing Stethoscope*. He is also a frequent contributor to medical periodicals.

William Beatty was born in Canada and received his B.A. (1951) and M.S. (1952) from Columbia. Since 1962 he has been Librarian and Professor of Medical Bibliography at Northwestern University Medical School. Mr. Beatty has written articles for library and medical journals and has contributed to books published in this country and England.